THE
INSULIN
RESISTANCE
FACTOR

Can't Lose Weight?
Can't Concentrate?
Can't Resist Sugar?
Could SYNDROME X Be Your Problem?

THE
INSULIN RESISTANCE FACTOR

A Nutritionist's Plan for Reversing the Effects of Syndrome X

ANTONY J. HAYNES

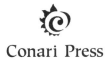

Conari Press

First U.S. edition published in 2012 by Conari Press,
an imprint of Red Wheel/Weiser, llc
With offices at:
665 Third Street, Suite 400
San Francisco, CA 94107
www.redwheelweiser.com

Published by arrangement with HarperCollins Publishers Ltd

First published by Thorsons 2004

10 9 8 7 6 5 4 3 2 1

© Antony Haynes 2004

Antony Haynes asserts the moral right to be
identified as the author of this work

ISBN 978-1-57324-549-4

Printed and bound in Great Britain by
Clays Ltd, St Ives plc

For Bharti and Ben

Contents

Introduction

Why should I read this book?

- Do you always struggle with your weight despite watching what you eat?
- Do you store most of your body fat around your middle?
- Do you always crave sugary or starchy foods?
- Do you have a poor memory or concentration and get a "fuzzy" brain, especially after eating?
- Do you regularly feel tired or lethargic even if you've had a good night's sleep?
- Do you have high blood pressure or high cholesterol?
- Do you have a history of heart disease or diabetes in your family?

If your answer is "yes" to one, two, or more of these questions you may well have an imbalance of a hormone in your body called insulin. And you are not alone. As many as four out of every five people have some degree of what is known as Insulin Resistance. Most of us aren't even aware of it and, generally speaking, it is only the 22 to 25 percent of the population who have full-blown Insulin Resistance who are more likely to get a proper diagnosis.

 A staggering 80 percent of the population have some degree of Insulin Resistance, 22 to 25 percent of which have full-blown Insulin Resistance

What is Insulin Resistance?

Insulin Resistance, also known as Syndrome X and the Metabolic Syndrome, is a condition that occurs when, for a variety of reasons, your body makes too much insulin.

Insulin is a powerful hormone secreted by the pancreas in order to control the way the body stores and uses carbohydrates in the body. Under normal conditions, insulin is produced within moments of blood glucose levels increasing, which occurs after we eat something. In simple terms, its purpose is to enable the muscles and other tissues to take up the glucose they require for activity and keep blood sugar levels to an acceptable level by storing any excess glucose for future use. However, for a variety of reasons—which, of course, we'll look at in detail—this mechanism can become faulty, with the result that some tissues become resistant to the effects of insulin and the pancreas has to produce more insulin to get the blood glucose level down. This has many important implications for your metabolism and your general health—in essence, it makes you overweight and tired, and it dramatically increases your risk, first of heart disease and then of type II diabetes. If left untreated, Insulin Resistance will often lead to type II diabetes.

 Insulin Resistance is also known as Syndrome X and the Metabolic Syndrome.

The good news is that whatever degree of Insulin Resistance you may have, you can completely reverse it by following the Insulin Factor Plan. This means that you will:

▼ Lose weight safely and permanently
▼ Feel energetic and alert
▼ Stop feeling tired or dizzy before or after meals
▼ Improve your memory and concentration
▼ Stop craving sugary and starchy foods
▼ Stop digestive problems from causing bloating, pain, constipation, etc.

- ▼ Slow down your body's aging process—look younger for longer!
- ▼ Lower cholesterol and high blood pressure
- ▼ Improve fertility and, if you are a woman, reduce your chance of developing PCOS (Polycystic Ovary Syndrome)
- ▼ Lower your risk of getting heart disease and cancer
- ▼ Alleviate inflammatory diseases such as arthritis and gout
- ▼ Never get type II diabetes

In short, you'll feel healthy, energetic, and ready for anything—it will dramatically improve your quality of life!

How do I get started?

The Insulin Factor Plan is not a one-solution-fits-all program because there are a range of imbalances that together or individually cause Insulin Resistance, and there are also different degrees of Insulin Resistance. With the help of questionnaires throughout the book you will be able to identify what degree of Insulin Resistance you have and which imbalances are causing it. Once you have pinpointed your imbalances—some of you will only have one or two, while others may need to address them all—you can turn to the end of the book and find out how to put together your personal plan of action. Generally speaking, you will need to make changes to your diet, take particular nutritional supplements, and look at your lifestyle. The Insulin Factor Plan will help you with all three. You will of course need to commit yourself to making these changes, but the fact that you have this book and are already reading it is a very positive first step. While Insulin Resistance doesn't happen overnight, it can take only a few weeks before you notice an improvement in your symptoms. However, you also need to be patient because it will take an average of six months to permanently rebalance your insulin levels. Also, the more weight you need to lose the longer you will need to allow.

Medical conditions

Balancing insulin and glucose and eating a healthy diet is something that everybody would benefit from, so the Insulin Factor Plan should complement any medical treatment you are receiving. However, you should always check with your doctor before embarking on any dietary or lifestyle changes, particularly if you are taking any medication. This is because the improved diet and lifestyle may alter your required dosage.

To help keep your motivation high, keep returning to the list of all the health benefits that will be yours when you have balanced your insulin levels. Write them down or photocopy them and stick them up on your fridge or keep them in the front of your diary—wherever you will see them. Know that if you follow the Insulin Factor Plan you will not only turn your back on all the health problems but you will, in their place, enjoy all the benefits. Good luck, and enjoy!

Part One

What is Insulin Resistance?

1 Tell Me About Insulin Resistance

What is insulin?

Although we've been talking about Insulin Resistance you shouldn't think that insulin is really the bad guy in all of this. Even though it is a dangerous hormone when it is produced in excessive amounts, as in the case of Insulin Resistance, it is actually vital for the body to function normally and to control how the body uses and stores glucose. Glucose is what gives your muscles and other organs the energy to function. Too little insulin is also just as dangerous, if not fatal, as seen in people who have type I diabetes: they can't produce insulin so they need to regularly inject themselves with this hormone. Without these injections their blood sugar level would be too high, which has serious and indeed fatal consequences. So, as with many things in life, it is a question of balance—too much or too little insulin in the body are just as dangerous for your health.

 Too much insulin can make you overweight and tired, and increase your risk of heart disease and diabetes; too little insulin means high blood sugar levels which damages your internal organs.

What exactly does insulin do?

Insulin is one of many hormones in the body, and is also a protein. It is made in and secreted from cells in the pancreas called the Islets of Langerhans, named after the German pathologist who discovered them. The pancreas is one of the most important organs involved in digesting food and storing the nutrients in what you eat in your body's cells. To give you an idea of proportion, about 98 percent of the cells of the pancreas are devoted to digestion, with the Islets of Langerhans cells accounting for the remaining 2 percent. The cells in the Islets of Langerhans that produce insulin are called beta cells, or B-cells. There are also alpha cells, or A-cells, which produce glucagon, a hormone that raises blood glucose levels.

Insulin and carbohydrates

Insulin's main function is storing glucose from the bloodstream into cells. This first involves converting glucose released into the bloodstream from the digestion of foods into glycogen. The body only has a limited capacity to store glycogen—the primary stores of glycogen in the body are the liver and muscles—so all other glucose is then stored as fat, known as adipose tissue. People who have Insulin Resistance typically store this fat around their middles. Either way, insulin lowers the concentration of glucose in the blood.

Insulin and proteins

Insulin doesn't just determine what happens to the carbohydrates that we eat, it also plays an important part in the way that proteins are metabolized. During the digestive process, many proteins are broken down into amino acids, which are then transported into the bloodstream. Insulin promotes the transit of amino acids into the liver and muscle cells. In this way it is involved in storing proteins away in the body, just as it does carbohydrates. It also inhibits the breakdown of protein in muscle for fuel. This is because if insulin is present, the body concludes that there is adequate glucose available and there is no need to break down muscle proteins for energy.

Insulin and fats

Similarly, insulin also has command over how fats are handled in the body. It inhibits the release of fats from fat tissue. This means that insulin prevents the use of your fat for energy in a similar way to how it stops your body from breaking down proteins. Insulin also promotes the production of fatty acids in the liver, which increases the amount of fats (bad cholesterol and triglycerides) circulating in the bloodstream—a potential risk for heart disease when present in excess.

Essentially, what all this means is that insulin prevents the body from overly using itself up and breaking down structural proteins and fats, especially if you do not eat enough food. Obviously this worked well when we were hunter-gatherers—it meant the body did not begin breaking down its reserves at the first sign of hunger. These days, few of us go hungry for any length of time, so insulin's supreme ability to store glucose at fat for future use is not nearly as important. In fact, the modern diet that encourages high insulin levels means that the body stores more glucose as fat, and we are at greater risk of becoming overweight and obese.

How much insulin your body releases depends on what you eat

Under normal conditions, insulin is produced moments after we eat something, so insulin levels will always be higher after we eat than before. As our blood glucose levels increase, the pancreas secretes insulin into the blood and insulin then performs the storage roles described above. The rate at which the blood glucose level increases is primarily determined by the amount of carbohydrate you eat. The volume of amino acids (proteins) you eat also has an effect on insulin production but much less than carbohydrates. If you eat a portion of carbohydrates, for example, this raises your blood glucose more than if you ate the same amount of protein, resulting in more insulin being released to store the glucose away. Once the glucose and amino acids are stored away, levels of insulin reduce accordingly. In this way, insulin levels vary throughout the day depending on the food we eat.

 Carbohydrates raise blood sugar more than proteins. This means that your body produces more insulin when you eat carbohydrates than protein.

Insulin Resistance

If the body is continuously exposed to high levels of insulin, the insulin receptor cells in the liver, adipose (fat) tissue, and muscle start to become inefficient. The way insulin binds to the receptors in the liver, fat, and muscle tissues becomes partially blunted. In essence, this means some tissues in the body become resistant to the effects of insulin so that insulin is not able to carry out its normal role. The body recognizes that there is too much glucose in the bloodstream so the pancreas produces even more insulin to try and compensate. When your body is consistently producing high levels of insulin it is a sure indication that you are resistant to insulin, hence the term "Insulin Resistance." The pancreas will ultimately become exhausted and unable to produce the insulin needed to maintain optimal glucose levels, and this is when you become diabetic.

The harm Insulin Resistance does

We already touched on this in the introduction but it is worth looking at the subsidiary effects of Insulin Resistance in detail.

You may wonder why it is vital for the body to keep down glucose levels in the bloodstream. As much as we need glucose to function, glucose at too high a level leads to oxidation and this causes tissue damage. This is what happens in poorly controlled diabetes, which can lead to peripheral neuropathy, renal conditions, and cataracts. Because high blood glucose is so damaging to your health, your body will do everything it can to maintain normal glucose levels. The only means the body has to do this is with insulin. As you will see, the list of health conditions associated with Insulin Resistance is long and unpleasant:

Lay Description	Technical Term
Heart disease	Coronary Heart Disease (CHD)
Obesity	Body Mass Index (BMI) of 30 or over
Breast cancer	Breast Cancer
High blood insulin levels	Hyperinsulinemia
High blood cholesterol levels	Hypercholesterolemia
High blood pressure	Hypertension
Adult-onset diabetes	NIDDM (noninsulin-dependent diabetes mellitus)
Blood sugar problems	Dysglycemia
Polycystic ovary syndrome	PCOS
Gout	Hyperuricemia
Arthritis	Osteoarthritis
High blood fat levels	Hypertriglyceridemia or hyperlipidemia
Low good cholesterol	Low HDL
Impaired Glucose Tolerance	Impaired Glucose Tolerance
Low blood glucose	Hypoglycemia
Fuzzy head after eating carbs	Carbohydrate Sensitivity

What causes Insulin Resistance?

While your genes (see chapter 11) can be a contributory cause of Insulin Resistance—there is a higher risk of Insulin Resistance among people of South Asian origin—generally speaking there are numerous controllable factors that cause or exacerbate Insulin Resistance. The most significant one is related to body weight, or more specifically body over-fatness, especially around the middle. This is compounded by a sedentary lifestyle and the resulting lack of muscle tissue, by aging, stress, high blood pressure, and by excess consumption of refined carbohydrates, overprocessed food, saturated fat, and processed vegetable fat. Interestingly, digestive health also plays an important role. Obviously, with the exception of genetic factors and aging, many of these factors are under our control and we can take positive action. You can look at how these factors are playing a part in your health in chapter 3, with the Insulin Resistance questionnaire.

Contributory factors in Insulin Resistance

- High intake of sugar and refined carbohydrates
- Sedentary lifestyle
- Being overweight or obese (BMI over 30)
- Excess body fat around the middle (abdominal obesity)
- Stress
- High blood pressure
- A lack of vital nutrients
- Genetic factors
- Increased inflammation in the body
- A diet high in saturated fat
- A diet high in processed vegetable fat

Insulin Resistance results from the body's protective mechanism to prevent high blood glucose. Insulin Resistance is an extremely common problem that can cause disease and limit life span. There are many things that raise blood glucose (e.g. refined carbohydrates, sugar, stress) but just one that lowers it—insulin. Insulin Resistance is reversible if you make changes to your diet and lifestyle.

Summary of key points

- The food you eat directly affects your insulin levels
- Insulin profoundly affects carbohydrate, protein, and fat metabolism
- High levels of insulin are dangerous and contribute to heart disease
- Diet and lifestyle are the main causes of Insulin Resistance; there is no single genetic cause of Insulin Resistance.

2 Are Refined Carbs and Sugar the Bad Guys?

They're sweet, they're comforting, they give you an instant feel-good high—small wonder that so many of us keep on turning to refined carbohydrates and sugar. We're also surrounded by food products containing these instantly gratifying substances—soft drinks, chocolate bars, bagels, pasta, ice cream, candies to suck, chew, or swallow—and because the "fix" we get from them is sweet and addictive, we are tempted time and time again.

We have been refining foods for centuries, as far back as the ancient Pharaohs who also observed the dangers of excess carbohydrates, but never as intensively since the middle of the 20th century. Too busy, too tired, too dissatisfied, or too depressed, we are easily seduced by the promise of a quick sugar or carb high. So, you may not want to hear it but carbohydrates and sugars really are the bad guys, especially when it comes to Insulin Resistance and all of its indirect effects. Understandably, it is a message most people don't want to hear. We are consuming more sugar in our diets today than ever before. In the USA the average person eats their way through a staggering 195 pounds of sugar in a year. This equates to every American eating nothing except sugar every fourth day!

Captain Cleave on sugar

As early as the 1930s a British Royal Naval doctor, Captain Thomas Latimer Cleave, identified the dangers of refined carbohydrates and sugar. He observed the correlation between rising incidences of heart and bowel disorders, obesity, diabetes, varicose veins, dental decay, hemorrhoids, and related diseases with the underconsumption of dietary fiber and overconsumption of refined carbohydrates. Sailing around the world between different countries and communities, he observed that there was a close correlation between the degree to which a society's diet was refined with cereals, rice, and sugar plants, and the incidences of these diseases. For instance, tribal communities eating a traditional whole-food diet were free from these diseases, whereas tribal communities who had adopted a more refined diet were not. He continued to study the effects of refined foods on health, eventually publishing *The Saccharine Disease* in 1974.

The sugar–body fat connection

The single most significant cause of being overweight is eating too many refined carbohydrates, for example, white bread, bagels, white pasta, white rice, cookies, cakes, candy, and chocolate. It is virtually impossible to be obese on a natural food diet. It is very easy to overeat refined carbohydrates because they are a denser form of calories—an apple contains the same amount of calories as a single teaspoon of sugar. You could quite easily consume 10 teaspoons of sugar in a fizzy drink but you'd be hard pushed to eat 10 apples in one sitting! The best way to avoid being overweight is to avoid refined carbohydrates. The ultimate refined carbohydrate is white sugar.

The key difference between natural foods and refined sugars is that natural foods contain fiber, vitamins, minerals, and other nutrients, whereas sugar and refined carbohydrates do not. This is why sugar and refined carbohydrates are often referred to as empty calories. What is more, sugar and refined carbohydrates also deplete nutrients in the body when they are metabolized. For example, every time you eat white sugar, you deplete your zinc and chromium levels because your body needs zinc and chromium in order to make insulin.

Fat consumption and exercise play a part in weight control, but they are not as important as you may think. It is quite possible to lose weight by reducing refined carbohydrates and not making any changes to your fat consumption and exercise routine. However, the Insulin Factor Plan does still recommend moderate exercise and emphasizes the need for good-quality fats.

Sugar and diabetes

There is also a strong link between sugar and diabetes. This is because refined carbohydrates encourage the body to produce high levels of insulin, which ultimately exhausts the pancreas so it is unable to make enough insulin to control blood glucose, leading to diabetes.

Sugar and heart disease

Not only does sugar increase your risk of diabetes, but it also increases your risk of heart disease. Interestingly, sugar will actually start affecting the health of your cardiovascular system long before you ever get diabetes. This is because high levels of insulin, normally caused by a diet high in refined carbohydrates, exist for many years before you develop diabetes, and excess insulin is one of the most powerful causes of furred arteries, high cholesterol and blood fats, (triglycerides), and high blood pressure (see chapter 1, page 7). Insulin is as responsible for elevated bad cholesterol and blood fats as dietary fat. As you know, there is a strong link between high cholesterol and blood fats, and heart attacks and strokes.

Sugar and tooth decay

Of course, it will come as no surprise that sugar is also the main culprit when it comes to tooth decay.

Digestive problems

Refined carbohydrates are also behind many digestive problems, because they feed unwanted bacteria in the gut. The refined carbohydrates line the wall of the gut and enable bacteria to thrive and survive rather than pass on through. These bacteria contribute to a range of conditions from excess gas, appendicitis, inflammation of the gallbladder, and poor digestion of fats, abdominal bloating, foul-smelling stools, and even cystitis and interstitial cystitis.

The hostile bacteria cause inflammation in the gut provoking the immune system to produce molecules called cytokines. This is a normal self-defense mechanism. However, an excess of these immune defense molecules causes problems in the same way excess insulin causes problems. They can escape the gut and get into the blood-stream and disrupt the binding of insulin to its receptor cells. Research shows that these cytokines are a significant contributory factor to Insulin Resistance.

This is why the health of your digestive system is an important part of the Insulin Factor Plan.

 Surprisingly, the health of your digestive system plays an important part in reversing Insulin Resistance.

But if you are completely horrified at the idea of not being able to eat sugar again, don't panic! Firstly, it's more a question of cutting down on foods that contain refined carbohydrates, and secondly it really isn't as difficult as you think, particularly because there are supplements you can take to stop your cravings. Most of my clients who are hooked on sugary things are surprised at how easy it can be to give them up.

Summary of key points

▼ Refined carbohydrates including sugar really ARE the bad guys when it comes to your health, particularly regarding Insulin Resistance.

▼ Sugar has been identified as a main cause of weight problems, heart disease, high cholesterol, diabetes, tooth decay, and even digestive problems.

▼ To restore your health, it is more a question of cutting down on refined carbohydrates, not necessarily cutting them out completely. In any case, there are supplements to stop your cravings, so it is not just a question of your will power!

3 What's My Risk of Insulin Resistance?

In this chapter you can find out about your own risk of Insulin Resistance. The first thing you have to do is to work out your Body Mass Index (BMI) and then you can go on to further assess your risk of Insulin Resistance by answering a five-part questionnaire. We'll also have a brief look at interpreting the results of a proper Insulin Resistance blood test, in case you want to do this, because it will give you a clearer indication of what degree of Insulin Resistance you have. We'll also look in a little more detail at the major causes of Insulin Resistance in relation to your questionnaire results and which sections you should focus on in your Insulin Factor Plan.

Body Mass Index (BMI)

You do not have to be overweight to be insulin resistant. However, being overweight and having a high proportion of body fat are significant risk factors for Insulin Resistance and heart disease. For this reason, it is helpful to work out your Body Mass Index, or BMI. There are two groups of people for whom a BMI reading is not always helpful or accurate, namely

▼ Athletes and those of a muscular build: it may overestimate body fat.
▼ Older persons and others who have lost muscle mass: it may underestimate body fat.

Generally speaking, though, your BMI is a reliable indicator of your total body fat.

Work out your BMI by using the BMI table (see Resources, pages 186–7). If you need help with assessing your BMI number, please talk to your doctor, who can work it out for you.

My BMI Number:
Date:

Interpreting your result

If your BMI puts you in the overweight or obese bracket, you need to start thinking about losing weight. People who are overweight have a greater chance of developing conditions that are caused at least in part by Insulin Resistance—high blood pressure, high blood fats and cholesterol, diabetes, heart disease, strokes, and certain cancers. Even a small weight loss (just 10 percent of your current weight) will help lower your insulin and consequent risk of developing those diseases. You shouldn't try to lose weight overnight because crash dieting actually increases Insulin Resistance. Instead you should follow the Insulin Factor Plan as recommended in chapter 12, which will help you lose weight steadily and permanently.

Underweight:	less than 18.5
Normal weight:	18.5–24.9
Overweight:	25–29.9
Obese:	more than 30

Insulin Resistance questionnaire

Now that you have calculated your BMI, you are ready to complete the Insulin Resistance questionnaire. The questionnaire is not meant to be the definitive and most accurate method of assessing Insulin Resistance, although it certainly is a good guide.

While you may have already made up your mind that you have Insulin Resistance, the following questions should give you clarification. Importantly, most "yes" answers—other than those in the family history section—can be addressed successfully with the Insulin Factor Plan. Even if you only have a low risk of Insulin Resistance, the questionnaire will show you which aspects of your diet and lifestyle you need to keep an eye on. It is also useful for you to return to and see what progress you have made.

The Insulin Resistance questionnaire is made up of five parts:

1 Family and Health History
2 Signs and Symptoms
3 Dietary Factors
4 Lifestyle and Exercise
5 Lab Test Results (not essential, but explanations are given so you can understand your results).

Part one—family and health history

Scoring this part of the questionnaire

This is simple. You need to answer "yes" or "no" to each question, with the exception of the age question. Each "yes" answer is given a single point. In the age question, you score more the older you are, with a maximum of 3 and a minimum of 0.

Do you have now or have you ever had in the past:
1 A family history of diabetes (type II), heart disease, or strokes?
2 A family history of obesity or high cholesterol?
3 Type II diabetes (noninsulin dependent, adult-onset)?
4 High blood pressure (Hypertension)?
5 High blood sugar (Hyperglycemia)?

6 Low blood sugar (Hypoglycemia)?

7 Polycystic Ovary Syndrome (PCOS)?

8 Gout or arthritis?

9 Kidney stones?

10 A BMI of 30 or over?

11 Take the birth control pill (now, or for more than a year in the past)?

12 Exercise less than one hour a week?

13 Are you of South Asian, African, Polynesian, or Mexican origin?

14 Crash dieted to lose weight quickly?

15 What is your age? (60+ = 3, 50–59 = 2, 30–49 = 1, under 30 = 0)

Score out of 17 (women) =
Score out of 16 (men) =

Part two—signs and symptoms

Scoring this part of the questionnaire

Again, "yes" answers score one point, but please note that if your BMI is equal to or over 33 then you score one point four times for the weight-related questions.

Do you have now or have you ever had in the past:

1 Is your BMI 33 or more?

2 Is your BMI 30 or more?

3 Is your BMI 27 or more?

4 Is your BMI 24 or more?

5 Difficulty losing weight despite exercise and/or a calorie-controlled diet?

6 An addiction to carbohydrates/candy?

7 Inexplicable fatigue, tiredness, lack of energy?

8 Headaches, nausea, or fatigue that is alleviated by eating?

9 A feeling of always being thirsty?

10 Need to eat every 3 hours or less?

11 Irritable after 4 hours without food?

12 Sleepy or fuzzy-headed particularly after carbohydrate meals?

13 Suffer from afternoon fatigue?

14 Indigestion after meals?

15 Acne?

16 Physically unfit?

17 Hirsutism (excess facial hair or on the thighs)? (Women only)

18 Dry, flaky skin?

19 An earlobe crease in each ear?

20 Postural hypotension (your blood pressure drops when you stand up)?

21 *Arcus senilis* in your eyes? (This is a marking in the colored part of the eye, the iris, where there is a white circle within the circumference, usually at the top of the iris under the eyelid (11–1 o'clock), but sometimes in the lower part too (4–8 o'clock), and sometimes around the whole iris)

Score out of 21 (women) =
Score out of 20 (men) =

Part three—Diet

Scoring this part of the questionnaire

Each "yes" answer scores one point. Please note that if you smoke more than 15 cigarettes a day, then you score one point three times for the smoking-related questions. The same principle applies to the alcohol, water intake, and vegetable intake questions.

Do you now or have you ever in the past:

1 Eat refined carbohydrates (e.g. white bread, white rice, sugar)?

2 Eat hidden sugars in foods or drinks?

3 Regularly eat large meals?

4 Smoke more than 15 cigarettes a day?

5 Smoke more than 8 cigarettes a day?

6 Smoke cigarettes every day or more than 10 a week?

7 Drink caffeinated drinks (with or without sugar) (e.g. coffee or cola drinks)?

8 Drink more than four cups of tea a day (with or without sugar)?

9 Drink more than 2 units/glasses of alcohol a day?

10 Drink more than 4 units/glasses of alcohol a day?

11 Eat fried food more than once a week?

12 Eat barbecued food more than once a month?

13 Eat processed foods regularly, including microwave or oven meals?

14 Eat protein foods (e.g. fish, white meats, eggs, meats) fewer than 3 times a week?

15 Are you a vegan (no meat or dairy products)?

16 Drink more than two glasses of fruit or vegetable juice a day?

17 Seldom eat oily fish, nuts, and seeds? (see chapter 6)

18 Eat less than one portion of fresh vegetables a day?

19 Eat less than two portions of fresh vegetables a day?

20 Eat two meals a day or less?

21 Eat just one meal a day?

22 Drink less than 3 glasses of water a day?

23 Drink less than 5 glasses of water a day?

24 Drink less than 8 glasses of water a day?

Score out of 24 =

Part four—lifestyle and exercise

Scoring this part of the questionnaire

Each "yes" answer scores one point, except where indicated with regard to frequency of exercise. Exercise in this context means anything in which you are physically moving for at least 20 minutes at a time, including aerobic, stretching, or resistance work.

Are you now or have you ever in the past:
1 Regularly stressed or anxious?

2 A poor sleeper?

3 Always chasing appointments or deadlines?

4 Unable to relax without feeling guilty?

5 A person who has a persistent need for achievement?

6 Easily angered?

7 A sedentary person (e.g. office worker)?

8 A person who does anaerobic (e.g. weights only) and no aerobic exercise?

9 A person who exercises 3–4 times a week (score 1)?

10 A person who exercises 1–2 times a week (score 2)?

11 A person who exercises less than once a week (score 3)?

12 A very competitive person?

13 Irritable and impatient?

Score out of 16 =

Part five—Blood test results

Scoring this part of the questionnaire

Read through this section and answer any questions for which you have blood test results. Skip this section if you have not had a blood test done.

Do you currently have any of the following?

1 High-fasting insulin

2 High-fasting triglycerides

3 High triglycerides after a meal

4 Decreased HDL (good) cholesterol

5 Elevated LDL (bad) cholesterol

6 Elevated total cholesterol

7 Elevated systolic blood pressure (your first figure is over 139)

8 Elevated diastolic blood pressure (your second figure is over 89)

9 Elevated fibrinogen

10 Elevated PAI-1 (plasminogen activator inhibitor-1)

11 High uric acid (or gout)

12 Low Serum or Salivary DHEA (DHEA may have an inverse relationship with cortisol and insulin)

13 Elevated testosterone in women (acute hyperinsulinemia increases testosterone blood levels and suppresses SHBG synthesis) (women only)

14 Low levels of sex hormone binding globulin (SHBG) (women only)

15 Decreased testosterone (serum or saliva test) (men only)

Score out of 14 (women) =
Score out of 13 (men) =

If you have answered "yes" to any of the questions above, other than insulin itself, you should consider a fasting glucose and insulin test to rule out Insulin Resistance and diabetes. Also, make sure you discuss "positive" results with your healthcare provider. (See Resources for laboratory information.)

Your scores

Section five of the questionnaire determines whether you have Insulin Resistance or not, and to what degree. However, the sections one to four of the questionnaire help to quantify your risk and will show you which aspects of the Insulin Factor Plan you need to follow. The higher your score in the first four sections, the more advisable it is to have an Insulin Resistance test.

Use the chart below to write down your scores and add them up.

Total scores

1 Family and Health History	/17 (F)
	/16 (M)
2 Signs and Symptoms	/21 (F)
	/20 (M)
3 Diet	/24
4 Lifestyle and Exercise	/16
5 Blood Test Results	/14 (F)
	/13 (M)
	———
Total	**/92 (F)**
	/89 (M)

Interpreting the questionnaire

While your total score is perhaps the most important indicator of overall risk for Insulin Resistance, the individual parts also have relevance. Both are categorized according to risk in the table below.

	Your Scores	Low Risk (Stage 1)	Moderate Risk (Stage 2)	High Risk (Stage 3&4)
Taken as a whole (all 5 parts)	/92 (F) /89 (M)	22 or less	23–49	over 49
Taken as a whole (parts 1–4)	/78 (F) /76 (M)	16 or less	17–41	over 41
Taken section by section				
1 Family and health history	/17 (F) /16 (M)	4 or less 4 or less	5–8 5–8	over 8 over 8
2 Signs and symptoms	/21 (F) /20 (M)	5 or less 5 or less	6–12 6–12	over 12 over 12
3 Diet	/24	5 or less	6–13	over 13
4 Lifestyle and exercise	/16	4 or less	5–8	over 8
5 Blood test results	/14 (F) /13 (M)	4 or less 4 or less	5–8 5–8	over 8 over 8

The Insulin Resistance questionnaire indicates the degree of Insulin Resistance you may have. The following information clarifies your risk of Insulin Resistance, and will help you plan your dietary and lifestyle changes.

1 **Family and Health History:** Only two elements in this section can change (weight and age), so this is a relatively fixed score. This sets the scene for your risk, but does not determine it.

2 **Signs and Symptoms:** If you scored highly on this part of the questionnaire, together with a moderate risk total score or more, it suggests that you could be at a moderately advanced stage of Insulin Resistance, particularly if you are overweight. You need to follow all parts of the Insulin Factor Plan.

If you score highly on this section but only score a low risk on all other parts of the questionnaire, then consider taking the Adrenal Stress Profile saliva test and study chapter 9 on stress. You will also need to follow the dietary plan in chapter 13, and the Adrenal Support Supplement Program.

3 **Dietary Factors:** If you scored highly on this part but not on the others, this puts you at risk of being in the early stages of Insulin Resistance, and increases your risk of developing it in due course. Eating refined carbohydrates represents the single biggest risk factor for developing Insulin Resistance. This risk is more pronounced if you score highly in part 4, Lifestyle and Exercise. You need to concentrate on the dietary plan in chapter 13, and follow the Insulin Resistance Supplement Plan One.

4 **Lifestyle and Exercise:** If you score highly in this section only then is there a need to start becoming more physically active. Even if you are not overweight you could well be in the early stages of Insulin Resistance. Inactivity is a profoundly important risk factor for Insulin Resistance, especially if you've scored highly in part 3 of the questionnaire, Dietary Factors. You need to read chapter 10 and find out the most suitable exercise for you.

5 **Blood Test Results**: These give "hard" evidence of your current degree of Insulin Resistance, which is examined in more detail on pages 181–2. It is unlikely that a high score in this part would not be matched by high scores in other parts of the questionnaire. Don't worry if your test results score highly. It doesn't mean you can't change them—far from it. In fact, the blood tests are an excellent way to monitor your improvements when you implement the Insulin Factor Plan.

Improving your situation

Your total questionnaire score, for either four or five parts, represents your baseline score, which will improve when you begin to implement the Insulin Factor Plan. Please redo parts 2 to 4 or 2 to 5 inclusive (not part 1, unless you have lost weight and are a year older) one month after you begin any changes in diet, nutrition, and exercise to see the reduction in your scores. This is a good way of monitoring how you are doing, and will hopefully encourage you to keep going. If your score does not go down at all, please review chapter 12, which provides you with the model of how to reverse Insulin Resistance, and double check that you have gone through the action steps and checklists. If, within another month, there is still no change, it would be best to go and see a qualified nutritionist (see Resources).

There are many other questionnaires in this book but the Insulin Resistance questionnaire is the most important. Keeping your results of the questionnaires in mind, let's now take a look at the six major causes of Insulin Resistance and how your questionnaire results tie in with them.

The six major causes of Insulin Resistance

There are six major causes of Insulin Resistance and your results from the questionnaires will show you how much of a contributor each one is to you.

1 **General diet:** eating too many refined carbohydrates and over-processed foods (this includes low nutrient levels and an imbalance in dietary fats—see chapters 5–8)
   Measured by the Diet Questionnaire

2 **Sedentary lifestyle:** lack of physical activity and exercise, and lack of muscle (see chapter 10)
   Measured by Exercise and Lifestyle Questionnaire

3 **Weight:** being overweight and/or having an elevated BMI (see this chapter)
Measured by BMI calculation, observation, and body composition measurements

4 **Stress:** abnormal stress hormones (cortisol and DHEA) have a negative effect on Insulin Resistance (see chapter 9)
Measured by Stress Questionnaire and adrenal hormone saliva test

5 **Lack of nutrients:** chromium, magnesium, essential fats, other nutrients (trace minerals, minerals, vitamins), including antioxidants (see chapters 6, 7, and 8)
Measured by Diet and Signs and Symptoms Questionnaires and blood tests

6 **Genetic influence**: a family history of diabetes, heart disease, and obesity and being of South Asian, African, Polynesian, or Mexican origin (see chapter 11)
Measured by Family and Health History Questionnaire

The Insulin Connection

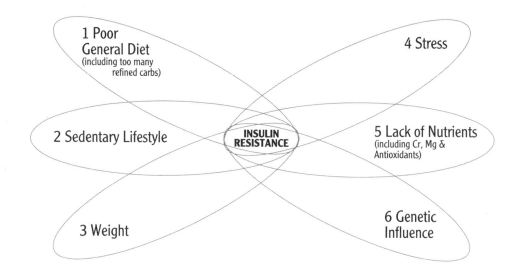

Age and insulin

Whatever your ethnic origin, your risk of Insulin Resistance increases as you get older. If you remain active, do gentle exercise to reduce loss of muscle mass, reduce the amount of calories you eat but increase the quality of your nutrient intake (as we age we become less efficient at digesting food), your age will not work against you and you will also find that you age more slowly.

However, it is also true that Insulin Resistance is becoming increasingly common in younger and younger people and a person's chronological age is a less obvious risk factor than it once was. In actual fact, people who develop Insulin Resistance as early as the late teens and early twenties have a prematurely aged metabolism—they have the metabolism you'd expect to see in someone at least twice their age. Don't worry if this sounds like you. Not only will the Insulin Factor Plan put your insulin and glucose levels back on track but it will also help you take years off your body's biological age—the best kind of side effect!

See Resources on pages 181–2 for help interpreting your Insulin Resistance Blood Test.

If you have done a blood test and know what degree of Insulin Resistance you have, turn to the Resources on pages 181–2. However, without a blood test you can still get a good idea about what degree of Insulin Resistance you have, and take the appropriate action as outlined below. Your questionnaire scores will reflect a low, moderate, or high risk of Insulin Resistance, which correlate with the different stages of Insulin Resistance that would be determined by the blood test.

Low Risk—Stage 1

You are insulin sensitive, and insulin levels fluctuate depending on food and drink intake, but you have normal fasting insulin and glucose levels. This does not mean you are free of symptoms, because you can put on weight if you eat too much, but this is not a dramatic or rapid process. You can also get symptoms of low blood sugar after eating a sugary meal like a big baked potato, because your insulin works well and is stimulated in large amounts by the high-sugar potato and consequently stores glucose into liver, muscle, and fat cells rapidly, resulting in "postprandial hypoglycemia." At this stage your blood test results would all be normal.

Action: Follow the Insulin Factor Diet Plan and Insulin Resistance Supplement Plan One

Moderate Risk—Stage 2

Your fasting insulin is still normal, as is your glucose. However, you can gain body fat more easily in this stage, and your fasting triglycerides (blood fats) would be elevated and the good cholesterol (HDL) low.

Action: Follow the Insulin Factor Diet Plan and Insulin Resistance Supplement Plan Two

High Risk—Stage 3

Your fasting insulin is elevated, as it is after eating, the triglycerides (blood fats) are high too, and the HDL is low, and, generally, you are overweight, especially around your middle.

Action: Follow the Insulin Factor Diet Plan and Insulin Resistance Supplement Plan Three

High Risk—Stage 4

Your scenario is the same as for stage 3 above, except that your fasting blood glucose is a little too high.

Action: Follow the Insulin Factor Diet Plan and Insulin Resistance Supplement Plan Three

Stage 5

At this stage you would technically be diabetic because your blood glucose would be too high.

Action: Follow the Insulin Factor Diet Plan and follow doctor's drug prescription. Supplements may be appropriate but should be recommended by a qualified nutritionist working with your doctor.

So, now you know your risk of Insulin Resistance. However, before you get going with the Insulin Factor Plan you need to take a closer look at the diet and lifestyle influences that will really make a difference to the speed at which you reverse Insulin Resistance. These are the two main areas of change that you will form part of your Insulin Factor Plan and getting to grips with them will make it much easier for you to succeed.

Summary of key points

▼ A high Body Mass Index (BMI) is a significant, independent risk factor for Insulin Resistance.

▼ The six major causes of Insulin Resistance are:
  1 Eating too many refined carbohydrates and overprocessed foods
  2 Sedentary lifestyle
  3 Being overweight
  4 Stress
  5 Lack of nutrients
  6 Genetic influence.

▼ Age is not a specific risk factor, but an associated one for Insulin Resistance.

▼ Insulin Resistance in younger people indicates an accelerated biological age.

▼ There are degrees of Insulin Resistance and these help to distinguish appropriate dietary and exercise recommendations.

Part Two

Let's Take a Look
at Diet

4 How Your Digestion Affects Insulin

Digestive problems are a hidden cause of Insulin Resistance. This is mainly because as much as 70 percent of the body's immune system is located within the gut, and if your gut immunity is taxed the gut is flooded with cytokines—if you remember these are immune messengers—and in large quantities these blunt receptors for insulin in your body. This means insulin becomes less effective at storing glucose away so the body produces more insulin to compensate. For example, this is why, if you have a food intolerance, you can have difficulty in losing weight: your immune system is battling with a perceived threat and, in producing cytokines to fight it, interrupts the usual efficient function of insulin.

It's not just food intolerances that cause an immune reaction in the gut. Yeasts, such as candida albicans, unfriendly bacteria, parasites, and maldigestion trigger cytokine activity as well. Poor diet is a major culprit because not only does it not provide adequate nutrients for optimal immune function but it creates an environment within the gut that favors and feeds unwanted bugs.

The other thing that causes or exacerbates the likelihood of both gut problems is stress. Stress directly weakens immunity within the gut, thereby leading to an inability to distinguish friend from foe (i.e. overreacting to an everyday food) and prevent the colonization of unwanted bugs.

Digestive problems are extremely common because the typical western diet is high in refined foods and we have lifestyles that expose us to high levels of stress.

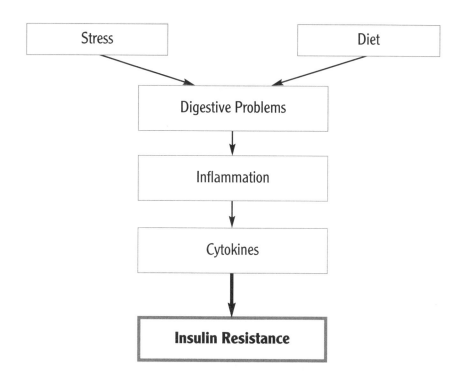

Gut Health Questionnaire

Answer "yes" or "no" to the following questions. Each "yes" answer is given a single point. Your total score will help you determine the likelihood of your digestive system contributing to Insulin Resistance.

Do you *regularly* (every few days) have:
  1 Indigestion or heartburn?
  2 Bloating after meals?
  3 Nausea?
  4 Excess gas and wind?
  5 Abdominal pain?
  6 Cramps?
  7 Irregular bowels?
  8 Diarrhea?
  9 Constipation (fewer than one motion per day)?
10 Hemorrhoids?
11 Known or suspected food intolerances?

12 Antibiotics?

13 Painkilling medications (e.g. aspirin or ibuprofen)?

14 Yeast or candida overgrowth?

15 Parasite or gut bacterial infections?

16 Food poisoning?

17 More than 14 units of alcohol per week?

Score out of 17 =

If you have any one of these **regularly** then your digestive health needs attention. If you've scored more than 5 then it almost certainly means it is compromising your Insulin Resistance, and warrants immediate action. If you have a pattern of any of these symptoms after eating specific foods then this suggests you have a food intolerance and this could be affecting your insulin sensitivity. It would be worth your while eliminating the suspected culprit food for a trial period of four weeks to see if your symptoms improve.

To address any digestive problems start the Insulin Factor Diet Plan and the Gut Supplement Plan rather than the Insulin Resistance Supplement Plan. It may take a number of weeks to reduce your questionnaire score, and only when you have reduced the score to 4 or less, and the symptoms are less regular, should you start following any of the Insulin Resistance Supplement Plans.

Summary of key points

▼ 70 percent of your immune system is located in the gut.

▼ Gut problems almost always involve the immune system.

▼ Immune system reactivity produces cytokines.

▼ Gut cytokines travel to the bloodstream and blunts the action of insulin.

▼ Food intolerances play an important role in the production of cytokines in the gut.

▼ Invariably, if you have Insulin Resistance and gut problems too, you need to address the latter first.

5 Carbs and Proteins—Your Key to Reverse Insulin Resistance

The Insulin Connection

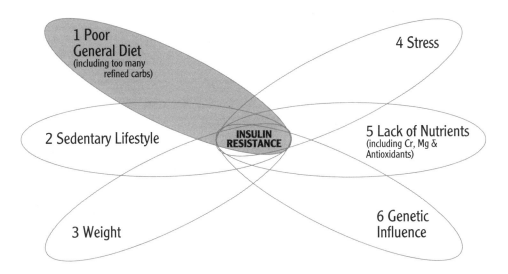

1 Poor General Diet (including too many refined carbs)

4 Stress

2 Sedentary Lifestyle

INSULIN RESISTANCE

5 Lack of Nutrients (including Cr, Mg & Antioxidants)

3 Weight

6 Genetic Influence

Mixed messages

With all this discussion about refined sugars and carbohydrates you may be wondering if you should still be eating them, especially because we are bombarded on a daily basis with conflicting opinions and information on what we should and should not be eating. First we are told that "fat is bad," then it's carbohydrates. What are we to do—not eat either? And how can we do that when we've been told that too much protein isn't good for us either? It's hardly surprising there are a lot of confused people.

What the headlines—and often the articles themselves—fail to explain is that there are good and bad fats, good and bad carbs, and good and bad proteins, all of which should ideally be eaten in balance with each other for optimum health. They also make an assumption that we are all the same, which is evidently not the case because each of us requires a different balance of nutrients to achieve good health. Take twins for example. They can have up to a twenty-fold difference in needs for some nutrients.* Imagine how different it could be between people who are not related!

To help you start to get to grips with some useful nutritional facts, this chapter looks at carbohydrates and fiber, the Glycemic Index, and then proteins. Lastly you'll find out what proportions of carbs and protein you should eat to reverse Insulin Resistance.

There are two questionnaires to help you figure out what kind of carbs and proteins you are eating. The carbohydrate questionnaire is the first.

The Carbohydrate Questionnaire

Scoring the questionnaire

Each "yes" answer scores 1 point.

Do you regularly:

1 Eat sugar or hidden sugars in food or drink?
2 Eat packaged foods such as breakfast cereals?
3 Eat white flour products (e.g. bread, pasta, cookies, cakes) and/or white rice more than 5 times a week?
4 Crave sweet foods?
5 Smoke cigarettes?
6 Drink more than 2 glasses of wine or beer a night?
7 Drink more than 3 cups of tea a day?
8 Drink more than 2 cups of coffee a day?
9 Drink fizzy drinks on most days?
10 Feel dizzy or irritable after 3 hours without food?

---

* Dr. Roger Williams, *The Wonderful World Within You: Your Inner Nutritional Environment.*

11 Get nauseous if you go without food, especially in the morning?

12 Get the shakes if you go without food for too long?

13 Get headaches if you miss a meal?

14 Need to eat frequent meals?

15 Urinate a lot during the day and night?

16 Have excessive thirst?

17 Have cold hands and feet?

18 Get tired?

19 Get anxious and stressed?

20 Work harder than most people?

21 Wake up in the night feeling hungry?

22 Are you addicted to carbohydrates/sweet foods?

Total Score =   /22

Interpreting the questionnaire

A high score in this questionnaire means you consume too many refined carbohydrates and this contributes to and increases your risk of Insulin Resistance. As you make changes to your diet, you should see your score reduce. Reading this chapter will help you understand why the wrong carbs are the major cause of Insulin Resistance.

0–5   Excellent! Keep your carb balance at this level. If you scored 5 or just under, see if you can score even lower by following the Insulin Factor Plan.

6–10 This suggests you have a blood sugar problem, which is caused by your diet. To resolve this as swiftly as possible you should follow the Insulin Factor Diet Plan and the Insulin Resistance Supplement Plan One.

11–15 Too much! This strongly indicates a blood sugar and insulin problem, and that your diet is the major culprit. You need to follow the Insulin Factor Diet Plan and the Insulin Resistance Supplement Plan that your Insulin Resistance Questionnaire indicated in chapter 3. You should also redo this questionnaire in four weeks' time to check your progress.

16+   Way too much! There's no doubt that your diet is a significant causative factor in your Insulin Resistance. You may benefit from doing the Insulin Resistance Blood Test. You need to follow the Insulin Factor Diet Plan and the Insulin Resistance Supplement Plan that your Insulin Resistance Questionnaire indicated in chapter 3. You also need to consider testing and balancing your adrenal hormones (see chapter 9). Use the questionnaires to monitor your progress. After four or five weeks, if there is no marked improvement despite changing your diet you should see a qualified nutritionist (see Resources).

Carbohydrate groups

Most foods actually contain a mixture of carbohydrates, proteins, and fats, and it's rare for any food to contain only one of these macronutrients. Some foods are dominant in carbohydrates, some dominant in protein, and some in fat. Carbohydrate-dominant foods consist of cereals, grains, starchy vegetables, and fruits. Legumes (beans and pulses) also contain predominantly carbohydrates even though they are often referred to as a protein food. Meats, fish, poultry, and eggs have little or no carbohydrate content, while dairy products can contain the carbohydrate lactose (milk contains more than hard cheese) and soy products can contain carbohydrates, depending on the type (e.g. tofu, soymilk, tempeh). Nuts and seeds have little or no carbohydrate (cashews contains the most, with 18 percent of its weight as carbs). Nonstarchy vegetables also contain some carbohydrates but in much smaller amounts than their starchy counterparts.

The most simple carbohydrates are known as simple sugars or monosaccharides. These are the fundamental building blocks of carbohydrates, just as the amino acid is the building block for proteins. When you eat a simple sugar or refined carbohydrate it requires little or no digestion and is absorbed quickly into the bloodstream. This elicits a rapid and excessive insulin response, and it is for this reason that refined carbs are so bad for you. The human body is not designed to handle REGULAR intake of refined carbohydrates with impunity.

 Refined carbs and simple sugars require little or no digestion and provoke a rapid and excessive insulin response. This is why they are so bad for you.

A system has been devised to measure how rapidly different carbs affect your blood glucose. This is called the Glycemic Index, which is a measure of the amount of insulin the body needs to produce to lower the glucose levels after eating that food. The higher the GI the more insulin is produced.

The Glycemic Index and Load

The Glycemic Index (GI) is a numerical system of measuring how fast a carbohydrate triggers a rise in circulating blood sugar—the higher the number, the greater the blood sugar response. So a low GI food will cause a small rise, while a high GI food will trigger a dramatic spike. A GI of 70 or more is high, a GI of 56 to 69 inclusive is medium, and a GI of 55 or less is low.

The Glycemic Load (GL) is a relatively new way to assess the impact of carbohydrate consumption. It takes the Glycemic Index into account, but gives a fuller picture than the Glycemic Index alone. A Glycemic Index score tells you only how rapidly a particular carbohydrate turns into sugar—but it doesn't tell you how much of that carbohydrate is in a serving of a particular food (i.e. the GI is a qualitative measure, whereas the GL is a quantitative measure). You need to know both things to understand a food's effect on blood sugar. The carbohydrate in watermelon, for example, has a high GI, but there isn't a lot of it, so watermelon's Glycemic Load is relatively low. A GL of 20 or more is high, a GL of 11 to 19 inclusive is medium, and a GL of 10 or less is low. Foods that have a low GL almost always have a low GI. Foods with an intermediate or high GL range from very low to very high GI. There is a detailed table in the Resources section showing the GI and GL of common foods.

The Glycemic Index and obesity

You may be surprised to know that it is not just the number of calories you eat that results in weight loss or weight gain. This is because calorie counting does not take into account the Glycemic Index and the hormonal response to food. Calorie counting can be helpful but should certainly not be the sole focus for weight loss. The reason why a low GI carbohydrate diet helps weight control is because it helps you feel satisfied after a meal and it both minimizes insulin levels after consumption and maintains insulin sensitivity.

Case Study: Carol

Resisting sugar is not just a matter of will power, however. I believe it is also linked to biochemistry and habit. When Carol came to see me some years ago she was in her early thirties and had been a member of overeaters anonymous for seven years. During this time she had not touched refined sugar and yet she still craved it. Sugar craving is sugar addiction, no matter which way you look at it. She was still addicted to sugar because she was having to use her willpower NOT to eat any. However, she still evidently had marked fluctuations in her blood glucose levels.

Based on her symptoms, a glucose tolerance test was recommended and the results were proof enough. Carol's blood glucose levels went up too high at first, into the mildly diabetic range, and then plummeted into the hypoglycemic range. She felt dreadful while the test was being performed—and remember this was after seven years of avoiding sugar. We did not measure her insulin and adrenal hormones at the time, but needless to say the insulin mounted a delayed response to the sugar shock and then was produced in high amounts, resulting in the sudden drop in blood glucose, at which time the adrenals would have kicked in to increase the level again. Carol was in stage 1 or stage 2 of Insulin Resistance, but was certainly not a full-blown case. There were also adrenal issues.

Carol was not eating enough protein by any means, with none whatsoever at breakfast. In addition, her diet as a whole was relatively high in carbohydrates, though these had a relatively medium to low Glycemic Index. I addressed her lack of protein by getting her to eat high BV (biological value) protein for breakfast, lunch, and dinner. She continued to eat some carbohydrates as well, so it was by no means a low or no carbohydrate diet at all. When she got into the habit of eating the protein foods her craving virtually disappeared. Her willpower enabled her to implement the new program, but it was the new program that gave her new-found freedom from her cravings. She has a motto, which I often use myself, "discipline equals freedom." The discipline to follow a program allows you to derive the benefits from that program.

 It is not how many calories you eat, but rather the type of calories you eat that causes weight gain.

What's the difference between simple sugars and starches?

Glucose (aka dextrose) is the best-known simple sugar. Sugars composed of two monosaccharide units are called double sugars or disaccharides, and these are found extensively in nature. Sucrose, also known as table sugar, is the best-known double sugar. When you eat sucrose, the enzyme sucrase splits it into the simple sugars glucose and fructose, which are then quickly absorbed into the body. More complex sugars, or polysaccharides, contain links of many simple sugars. Starch, for instance, contains polysaccharides, and are therefore known as complex carbohydrates. Plant starch requires much greater digestion and hence is absorbed much more slowly than less complex sugars like sucrose or glucose. As a consequence, starchy vegetables have a medium to low Glycemic Index.

Starchy vegetables

Some examples of starchy vegetables are given below:

Artichokes	Parsnip (cooked)
Beets	Potato
Carrots	Pumpkin
Corn	Sweet potato
Green peas	Turnip (cooked)
Leeks	Yam

Cooking transforms more complex carbs into more simple carbs. This means that the GI of raw starches is almost always lower than cooked starches.

Fiber foods

Just as starch slows down digestion, so too does fiber. Fiber makes you feel more full, which helps reduce appetite and slows the release of sugar into the bloodstream. It feeds friendly bacteria and carries toxins out of the gut, so unwanted bugs are less able to flourish.

Essentially, there are two kinds of fiber, soluble and insoluble. Soluble fiber absorbs much more water, toxins, and even cholesterol than insoluble fiber, and carries them all through the colon for elimination; insoluble fiber provides bulk but can irritate the gut lining, especially when eaten in excess. For example, oat bran, which is a rich source of soluble fiber, can lower cholesterol levels whereas wheat bran, a rich source of insoluble fiber, does not.

Rich sources of soluble fiber	Rich sources of insoluble fiber
Soluble	Wheat bran
Fruits	
Vegetables	
Legumes	
Oats	
Pectin	

Legumes—which contain plenty of soluble fiber—are a particularly useful source of carbohydrate in the diet. This is because they have a low Glycemic Index and are very insulin-friendly. Unfortunately, some people may find that legumes can cause excess gas, so introduce them gradually into your diet. If, however, the problem persists it may be due to a lack of digestive enzymes and you may need to either avoid them altogether or reduce the volume of legumes eaten and instead consume more starchy vegetables.

In some countries legumes are a staple; however, in the West they are not as common—with the exception of baked beans. However, instead of opting for denatured, often sugar-loaded, canned baked beans why not try some of the following:

Azuki beans	Chickpeas
Black beans	Green string beans

Haricot beans	Mung beans
Lentils/Split peas	Navy beans
Lima beans	Pinto beans

Grains

Starchy vegetables, legumes, and grains are the three main foods groups from which we derive the bulk of our carbohydrates. Fruit is also a high carbohydrate food. Of these groups it is grains that are most often refined and processed—and it is food processing that is largely to blame for the huge increase in refined, high Glycemic Index foods. The main staple foods around the world are wheat and rice. However, there is more to grains than just the big two. Below is a list of grains and, where appropriate, the sorts of foods that are made from them. Where possible, opt for the unrefined product—whole-wheat breads, whole-wheat pasta, unrefined breakfast cereals, brown rice, quinoa, millet grains, and so on.

Grains	**Food**
Wheat (white & brown)	Bread, pasta, breakfast cereals, cakes, cookies, couscous
Rice (white & brown)	Pasta, bread, cookies, crackers, ricecakes
Oats	Porridge, oatmeal bars, cookies
Rye	Bread, pasta, crackers
Barley	Bread, pasta, cereals
Millet	Bread, pasta
Buckwheat	Pasta, noodles
Bulgur	Tabouleh
Corn *	Tortilla chips, pasta, popcorn
Quinoa	Cereals
Polenta	

* Generally, corn is processed and refined

Fruit

While fruit contains many beneficial nutrients, such as antioxidants, vitamins, minerals, fiber, and water, as a food group, fruit is higher in carbohydrates and lower in protein and fat than any other. Fructose is the main carbohydrate in fruit, which is absorbed more slowly than glucose but still more quickly than complex carbs found in whole grains and legumes. For this reason you should be careful about how much fruit you eat. For the archetypal physically fit and lean individual, fruit will not be an issue, but the more insulin resistant you are, the more likely it is that you need to limit your fruit intake. If you have full-blown Insulin Resistance, you should only eat the lowest Glycemic Index fruits.

Higher GI fruits	Lower GI fruits
Banana	Blackberries
Dates	Blueberries
Figs	Cherries
Grapes	Grapefruit
Prunes	Raspberries
Raisins	Strawberries
Watermelon	

Limit carbohydrates, don't avoid them

If you have Insulin Resistance you should limit all carbohydrates, but not avoid them. However, you should avoid all *high* Glycemic Index foods. You can eat moderate to low Glycemic Index foods, such as many of the above grains in their whole form and in small amounts, although the more insulin resistant you are the fewer you should eat. Some people consider grains to be a primary cause of the Insulin Resistance phenomenon, and recommend an avoidance of all grains, both whole and refined. However, this is not practical for most people and can also cause health problems in the longer term. Instead of cutting out carbs altogether, concentrate on cutting out *refined* carbs from your diet and choose instead starchy vegetables and legumes as your main source of carbohydrate, and whole grains as a limited source—this cannot be emphasized enough.

Main sources of carbohydrate

Try to limit your carb intake to 40 percent of your diet, and within this 40 percent the following proportions:

Starchy vegetables	35%
Legumes (beans/pulses)	35%
Fruits	15%
Cereals/grains	15%

Why shouldn't I cut out carbs altogether?

Don't make the mistake of thinking that if low GI is good, no GI (i.e. eating no carbs at all) is better. Whatever degree of Insulin Resistance you have, it's made worse if you eat no carbs at all. Eating a very low carb diet for more than a couple of weeks can reduce the activity of your thyroid hormones, in particular the most active thyroid hormone, T3, or tri-iodo-thyronine. A low level of T3 can lead to fatigue, weight gain, and poor circulation. What's more, a low carb diet will also cause your blood glucose to drop and, when this happens, your brain stimulates the adrenals to raise blood glucose with cortisol, resulting in high cortisol levels. Independently of eating a low carb diet, high cortisol levels will actually reduce the thyroid hormone T3 and also increase Insulin Resistance (see chapter 9).

To make matters worse, chronically high cortisol levels trigger your body to break down muscle to provide your brain with glucose. Your muscles are the most metabolically active tissues in your body, so the less you have the more your metabolism will slow down.

A very low carbohydrate diet can result in weight loss in the first couple of weeks, but in the longer term can often damage your metabolism, lower your levels of the thyroid hormone T3, and tax your adrenals to an even greater extent. In short, a very low carb diet will make you more insulin resistant.

In short, what this all means is that while a very low carbohydrate diet can result in weight loss in the first week or so, in the longer term it can often damage your metabolism, lower your levels of the thyroid hormone T3, exacerbate Insulin Resistance, and tax the adrenals to an even greater extent. If you replace carbs with saturated fat, as advocated by the Dr. Atkins diet, you may feel better in the short term but it will not repair the damaged insulin receptors. This means that as soon as you stop the diet, you are likely to put weight straight back on again.

Serving size

How much carbohydrate you should eat in order to avoid stimulating too much insulin depends on the degree of Insulin Resistance you have. The greater the degree of Insulin Resistance you have, the less you should eat. This is not to say that if you do not have Insulin Resistance you can eat as much as you like or that if you have full-blown Insulin Resistance you should have none.

To give you an idea about the kind of serving size of carbohydrates that exist in carbohydrate foods here are some examples.

Starchy vegetables, legumes & grains

Food & serving size	Portion size
Carrots	1 large (3.5oz)
Corn	⅔ cup (3.5oz)
Leeks	½ cup (3.5oz)
Peas	½ cup (2.5oz)
Potato	1 medium, baked (3.5oz)
Pumpkin	½ cup (4.2oz)
Sweet potato (baked)	3.5oz
Oats	½ cup (4oz)
Quinoa	½ cup (3.5oz)
Rye bread	1 slice
Whole-wheat bread	1 slice
Brown rice	½ cup (2.5oz)
Ricecakes	5 thick cakes

Nonstarchy vegetables

Nonstarchy vegetables do not contribute to the carbohydrate content of a meal in the way that the starchy vegetables do, and they make an important contribution to the mineral, vitamin, and fiber content of your diet. Try to eat them fresh as possible because the fresher they are the more nutrients they will contain.

Here are some examples of nonstarchy vegetables and herbs:

Asparagus	Green beans
Bell peppers (green & red)	Kale
Broccoli	Lettuce
Brussels sprouts	Mangetout peas
Cabbage	Mushrooms
Carrots (raw)	Onions
Cauliflower	Parsley
Celery	Radish
Cilantro	Scallions
Cucumber	Spinach
Eggplant	Sprouts
Endive	Watercress
Garlic	Zucchini
Ginger	

Cravings and addictions

Sugar and refined carbohydrates are the most common addictions in the world—and with good reason. Firstly, and there's no denying it, they taste great! Secondly, because the brain relies on glucose to function properly, it sends signals to you to eat something sweet or starchy when it senses a drop in your blood sugar levels. Blood sugar fluctuations are extremely common and so are sugar cravings by default. However, every time you eat something sugary your body also produces more insulin to stop your blood sugar from getting too high. Your blood sugar drops again and then of course your brain tells you to eat more. This can easily become an addictive cycle. It's no coincidence that the symptoms of Insulin Resistance are also symptoms of blood sugar fluctuations, for example irritability, fatigue, sugar blues, moodiness, poor concentration, and, of course, sugar cravings. If you eat carbohydrates that release glucose more slowly into the bloodstream, insulin will not be produced in such large quantities and your blood glucose will be more stable. The immediate effect of this is to reduce the symptoms above and the longer term effect is to reverse Insulin Resistance. You might think that giving up sugar is impossible, that your cravings for it would be too intense. Don't worry, the Insulin Factor Plan directly addresses cravings and there are particular supplements, such as Glucobalance, that will help reduce them as well. It will actually be a lot easier than you think.

Summary of dietary recommendations for carbohydrates

▼ Eat only whole, natural carbohydrates and vary these to obtain a mixture of fibers.

▼ Avoid sugar and refined carbohydrates, where possible.

▼ Eat moderate to small portions of all types of carbohydrates at any meal.

▼ Eat small portions of carbs at each meal.

▼ Choose lower Glycemic Index carbs (see Resources).

Introducing protein

We'll now look at proteins and amino acids, the building blocks of protein, and why protein is so important to help reverse Insulin Resistance. First of all you need to complete the Protein Questionnaire to see if you are eating enough of the right proteins to support your metabolism.

The Protein Questionnaire

As with all the other questionnaires, the lower your score the better.

Scoring the questionnaire

Each "yes" answer scores 1 point.

Are you currently:

1 Vegan (i.e. no meat, eggs, or dairy)?
2 Lactovegetarian (dairy products only)?
3 Ovovegetarian (eggs only)?
4 Eating protein foods only once a day maximum?
5 Eating protein foods less than once a day?
6 Consuming the majority of your food from carbohydrate foods?
7 Experiencing blood glucose or insulin problems?
8 Overweight?
9 Depressed?
10 Exercising hard more than five hours a week?
11 Did you score over 15 on the Adrenal Stress Questionnaire (see chapter 9)?

Interpreting the questionnaire

The higher your score, the more need you to change the kind and quantities of proteins you eat. Here is what the scores indicate.

0–3 If you score 1–3, this isn't too bad, but you should still follow the Insulin Factor Diet Plan. If you are vegetarian, then it is recommended you consider using protein powders (see chapter 14).

4–7 This score strongly suggests you need to consume more protein to help you reduce insulin, balance blood glucose levels, and support your adrenals. The meal suggestions in chapter 13 will help you do this. If you are vegetarian, then you should seriously consider using protein powders (see chapter 14).

8+ You are in urgent need of increased protein intake, and probably amino acid supplements too. You may also require stomach acid support, as well as digestive enzymes, in order to maximize the benefit from eating more protein. See chapter 4 for more information on gut health. Again, if you are vegetarian, you should seriously consider using protein powders (see chapter 14).

Protein

The word protein is derived from the Greek word "protos" meaning primary or first. This is because it was the first nutrient to be discovered. Proteins are made by linking together various amino acids (more than 22 different kinds of amino acids are known). Enzymes, muscle, and egg white are examples of protein. Proteins are found in virtually every tissue in the body and amino acids play a major role in nearly every chemical function. Protein is therefore the single most important element in the diet.

However, just as there is confusion over carbohydrates, so there are also misunderstandings about protein, which we will look at.

Functions of proteins

Protein carries out many functions in the body. Hormones are derived from proteins, as are enzymes. Everything from bone, skin, ligaments, tendons, hair, nails, and teeth, to muscles and cell membranes, are made from protein. Glands and organs are also made from protein. The very structure of our DNA and genes are proteins. Hemoglobin is a protein. Half the dry weight of the body is protein. Your body needs amino acids to rebuild proteins, which it must do on a daily basis. However, the body cannot store amino acids, so it must obtain them from your diet. If you eat poor-quality proteins, or do not get enough, then your body is unable to properly rebuild and renew tissues.

Protein facts

Your gut lining replaces itself every four days, your skin rebuilds itself in 28 days and your whole blood supply turns over in 90 days. It takes just six weeks for every molecule in your bones to be replaced and six months for every molecule in your muscles to be replaced.

When you are trying to reverse any metabolic disorder, it is vital you get the highest-quality proteins, and this couldn't be truer than with Insulin Resistance. This is because high-quality proteins balance blood glucose levels and thereby reduce insulin and Insulin Resistance.

Amino acids

Proteins are made up of amino acids. There are 22 of these, of which some are essential and some nonessential. The body cannot make the essential amino acids from others and therefore they must be provided in our diet. There are also a number of amino acids the body normally makes for itself by converting the essential proteins you eat. However, some people may either not eat enough total protein or be unable to convert the proteins they've eaten properly. This small group of amino acids are called "semi-essential" amino acids, even though they are actually essential for some. If you are vegetarian, it is likely that these so-called "semi-essential" amino acids will actually be essential, and that you will need to obtain them from your diet.

Essential amino acids
Isoleucine
Leucine
Lysine
Methionine
Phenylalanine
Threonine
Tryptophan
Valine

Semi-essential amino acids
Arginine
Carnitine
Histidine
Taurine

Biological value

You can tell the quality of a protein from its amino acid composition—the wider range of essential amino acids a protein contains the higher the quality of the protein. Just as there is a qualitative measure for carbohydrates, as we saw with the Glycemic Index, there is also a qualitative measure for proteins called the Biological Value (BV). When the Biological Value was developed whole egg was found to be the highest-quality protein, and was accordingly given a BV of 100. Since then only one other food has been found to have a higher BV than egg, namely whey protein. Depending on the quality of how it is processed, the BV varies from about 100 to 159. You'll find that whey protein is recommended for breakfast in the Insulin Factor Diet Plan and for good reason.

Here are the BVs of some protein foods and protein powders:

Whey protein (ion exchanged, cross-filtered)	159
Whey protein concentrate (lactalbumin)	104
Whole egg	100
Cheddar cheese	95
Cows' milk	91
Egg white (albumin)	88
Fish	83
Beef	80
Chicken	79
Casein (from dairy)	77
Soy	74
Rice	59
Wheat	54
Almonds	52
Beans (haricot)	49
Yogurt	47
Hazelnut	45
Millet	33

To help you visualize the balance of amino acids and a food's BV, the graph on page 53 shows you the profile amino acids of egg protein. As you can see, an egg contains all the essential amino acids, hence its BV of 100.

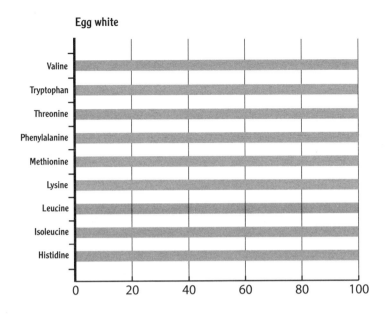

Egg white

In contrast, the graph below shows the essential amino acid profile of the protein in yogurt. As you will see the lowest amino value is tryptophan which is only 47 percent. The quality of a protein is determined by the lowest essential amino acid value, hence yogurt's BV is 47. This is because all the essential amino acids need to be present before the body can make something of them (i.e. when one is missing, the others cannot be used properly).

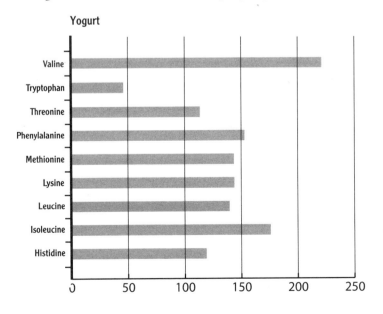

Yogurt

This is not to say that foods with a low BV are of no nutritional value. However, for a person with Insulin Resistance, foods with a BV of more than 75 play a key role in balancing blood glucose, which minimizes insulin and cortisol. When insulin is high, glucagon is low, and vice versa. Glucagon is the hormone that raises blood glucose when it is too low and helps sustain energy levels. So, by eating high BV protein foods you not only minimize insulin and cortisol but you also maintain good levels of glucagon.

Essentially, it's much easier to recognize a high BV protein food than it is to figure out the Glycemic Index of a carbohydrate. The protein foods with a BV of 75 or higher include: eggs, red meats (beef, pork, lamb, veal), poultry (chicken, turkey, game), fish (tuna, mackerel, salmon, sea bass, plaice, cod, haddock, sardines, etc.) and dairy (cheese and milk). The only vegetable food that comes close is soy—nuts, seeds, legumes, and grains are low BV foods. However, vegetarians should choose whey powder over soy because eating too much soy can lead to digestive, allergic, and hormonal problems. It is always better to choose fermented soy foods such as tempeh and miso.

Interestingly, the same proteins that body builders use are also the most suitable ones to help balance glucose, insulin, and cortisol as well. This is a key piece of information. This is because high BV proteins encourage muscle growth in the body as well as balancing blood glucose and minimizing insulin and cortisol. Of course, the more muscle you have, the more efficient your metabolism and the less fat you store.

Carb protein balance

The key to eating carbohydrates and proteins to reverse Insulin Resistance and, in fact, any type of blood glucose imbalance, is to eat the right quality and quantity of each. When you eat them together they have a different effect than when eaten alone. Protein slows down the digestion of carbohydrates and the rate at which glucose enters the bloodstream. This means that the impact of whatever carb you eat is reduced when you eat it with a high BV protein. As a general rule, you should eat twice as much low GI carbohydrate as you do high BV protein at a meal (i.e. eat a high BV protein at each meal). If you are very overweight or have stage 3 or 4 Insulin Resistance, you will need to reduce the amount of carbohydrate to protein eaten to about one and a half to one, or even less. When your BMI reduces to less than 30 (see chapter 3) you can slowly increase the amount of carbohydrates to two to one. I have used these principles at my clinic with consistent success.

 As a general rule, you should eat twice as much low GI carbohydrate as you do high BV protein at a meal.

How much should I eat?

The amount you eat is also important, because a large meal, even if it does contain insulin-friendly foods, still provokes a high insulin response. This is because the larger the meal the more nutrients there are to store away—and insulin is the storage hormone. It is far better to eat four or five smaller meals than two or three larger ones.

A typical ideal portion size for a meal would be something like a piece of fish the size of your palm, and about an inch (2.5cm) thick, two medium-sized boiled potatoes, three broccoli florets, and half a cup of steamed spinach. If you are overweight or have a more profound degree of Insulin Resistance, then you should have only one medium-sized boiled potato. Chapter 13 gives you plenty of meal suggestions in the right proportions.

Case Study: Martin

Martin, aged 36, came to see me in June 2003. His experience is relevant to the vast majority of people with imbalanced levels and functions of insulin and cortisol. He exercises four to five times a week and is physically fit. He is 6 feet 1 inch tall and weighs 168 pounds. He also watches what he eats. He was eating three meals and three snacks a day, and I noted that he ate a high BV protein at each meal, including a protein powder.

He was worried because he had recently changed his usual diet to be more vegetarian. Importantly, he hadn't increased the volume of food that he ate nor the GI of his carbs. He told me that in just three weeks he noticeably lost muscle, lost strength—as testified by the weight he could lift in the gym—and visibly increased his body fat. He also felt more tired. Even though he quickly changed back to his previous diet and a few weeks later his metabolism, weight, muscle, and energy levels were back to normal he couldn't understand the changes that had occurred. As you may guess, and as I explained to him, the key difference in Martin's diet was the BV of the proteins he ate. This is a classic example of how important high BV proteins are in controlling insulin and maintaining a healthy metabolism, and how much more difficult it is—but by no means impossible—for vegetarians to reverse Insulin Resistance than it is for an omnivore.

The healthiest BV foods

The best high BV protein foods you can eat are fish, lean white meats, and eggs, and, of course, whey protein powder. Red meats and cheese contain high levels of saturated fat, so it is best to eat them only once or twice a week. You'll find out why in chapter 6.

Summary of key points

▼ Carbohydrates raise insulin more than any other food, and some more than others.
▼ The Glycemic Index and Glycemic Load tell you how quickly and to what degree a carbohydrate food raises blood glucose and insulin.
▼ Choose moderate to low GI carbs to help balance blood glucose and insulin levels.
▼ Carbohydrates that contain natural fiber, particularly soluble, release their sugars more slowly into the bloodstream than carbohydrates stripped of their fiber (i.e. refined carbohydrates).
▼ Protein is essential for a multitude of functions, including building muscle and balancing blood glucose and insulin.
▼ Proteins consist of a number of amino acids which are essential, semi-essential or nonessential. The quality of proteins you eat are determined by the amount of essential amino acids they contain.
▼ The Biological Value (BV) of a protein is an indication of the essential amino acid content.

▼ Choose proteins with a BV of more than 75 at each meal to balance blood glucose, minimize insulin and optimize glucagon.

▼ Eating high BV proteins reduces the GI of carbs eaten at the same time.

▼ As a general guide, eat a ratio of 2 to 1 carbs to protein at every meal.

▼ Eat small regular meals.

6 What's So Essential About Essential Fats?

Most of us have spent years thinking that fat is bad for us, and while this is true of some fats there are actually others that are essential for our health. This chapter tells you about the good, the bad, and the ugly fats. The essential fats will play a key part in helping you reverse Insulin Resistance. As you'll remember from chapter 3, a poor diet is one of six major causes of Insulin Resistance. However, even if you change your diet and eat the correct balance of good carbs and proteins, if you are not eating enough essential fats you won't be able to reverse Insulin Resistance completely. But before we go into any more detail, see how highly you score in the Fats Questionnaire—are you eating enough of the right ones?

Fats Questionnaire

Scoring the questionnaire

Each "yes" answer scores one point.

Do you currently have:
1 Eczema or dry, flaky skin?
2 Rough skin?
3 A need to apply moisturizer to your body?
4 Excessive thirst?
5 Dry eyes?
6 Poor memory?
7 Poor sleep?
8 Loss of hair or dandruff?
9 Poor wound healing?
10 PMS or breast tenderness at any time? (women only)

11 Cravings for fatty foods?

12 Infertility?

13 Aching or sore joints or arthritis?

14 Depression?

15 Regular processed food including takeouts?

16 Eat fried food?

17 Eat red meat more than twice a week?

18 Eat nuts and seeds fewer than three times a week?

19 Eat fatty fish fewer than three times a week?

20 Eat dark green vegetables fewer than four times a week?

21 Add olive oil to your food fewer than three times a week? (excluding frying)

22 Nausea after eating fatty foods?

Score =   **/22 (women)**

Score =   **/21 (men)**

Interpreting the questionnaire

Essentially, the higher your score the more you need to change the kind of fats you are eating, because proper insulin function also relies on essential fats. (Please note, I use the terms "essential" and "good" fats interchangeably, though there is a technical difference between them.)

(Chapter 14 gives you detailed information about supplements, and what to do if you are vegetarian and cannot tolerate fish oil.)

0–3   This is a positive sign that your essential fatty acid balance is ideal or close to it. Carry on! You may still benefit from adding a fish oil (e.g. Super EPA) to your diet.

4–9   This is a fairly typical score, but typical is not ideal. You need to eat more essential fats as explained below, and follow Good Fat Supplement Plan A.

10–15   It's important you increase the amount of essential fats in your diet. It's more than likely that this imbalance is interfering with insulin activity. For example, eat oily fish three times a week, add nuts and pumpkin seeds to your diet and add olive oil to salads. You need to follow Good Fat Supplement Plan B.

16–21 You are almost certainly deficient in essential fats, and it is extremely likely that it is interfering with how well your insulin is working. You really need to start eating foods rich in the good fats, such as fish, nuts, and seeds. You need to follow Good Fat Supplement Plan C.

If you answered "yes" to question 22 about nausea, this also suggests you have a digestive problem—see chapter 4. Remember, you need to sort out your digestive problems before you focus specifically on Insulin Resistance. Do start eating more essential fats as advocated in the Insulin Factor Diet Plan but do not start any of the Insulin Resistance Supplement Plans. Instead focus on the Gut Supplement Plan in chapter 14.

Fats—the good, the bad, and the ugly

There are a number of different fats—some are vital for life, some are not, and some are downright bad for you. The naming of fats matches the structure of their molecules, hence we have polyunsaturated fatty acids (PUFAs), which are good; monounsaturated fatty acids (MUFAs), which are partly good; saturated fatty acids (SFAs), which are bad in excess; and trans fatty acids (TRANS), which are most definitely ugly. Let's start with the best fats—the essential fatty acids.

Essential fatty acids

Essential fatty acids (EFAs) are specific types of unsaturated fats that can only be obtained from the diet. They perform many vital roles in maintaining good health. The essential fats are divided into two families—the omega 3 and omega 6. Olive oil contains fats from another family of nonessential fats, called omega 9. The omega 3 and 6 oils are very delicate and deteriorate rapidly. Therefore, they are only found in fresh foods.

Essential Fatty Acid Group	Key Fatty Acids	Good Dietary Sources
Omega 3 family	Eicosapentaenoic acid (EPA), Docosahexaenoic acid (DHA), Alpha linolenic acid (ALA)	Salmon, mackerel, tuna, sardines. Present in human breast milk. Linseed oil & seeds (also known as flax), and pumpkin seeds. Small amounts in green leafy vegetables.
Omega 6 family	Linoleic acid (LA), Gamma linolenic acid (GLA), Arachidonic acid (AA)	Plant seed oils, e.g. sunflower, safflower, soy, corn/maize oils. Good sources of GLA are borage oil, evening primrose oil, blackcurrant seed oil. GLA is present in breast milk.
Omega 9 family	Oleic Acid (OA)	Olive oil (about 70% oleic acid). Also in nut oils (almond and walnut).

Generally speaking, foods contain a mixture of oils, but the table above shows only the predominant essential fat, with the exception of linseeds and pumpkin seeds. Pumpkin seed, for example, contains up to 15 percent of alpha linolenic acid (omega 3), 40–55 percent of linoleic acid (omega 6) fat and about 30 percent of oleic acid (omega 9). Because there are very few vegetarian sources of omega 3 essential fats, the linseed and pumpkin seeds have classified as omega 3 sources.

Functions of essential fats

Essential fats are made up of long carbon chains, some of which are bound together with double bonds. After digestion, essential fats are converted into even longer carbon chains of fats with more double bonds. It is these longer carbon chain fats that have many vital functions in the overall health of the body. Each omega family converts into a different longer carbon chains fat and they are vital for different functions—i.e. they cannot be used interchangeably.

Omega 3 family

Omega 3 essential fats help:

▼ Improve Insulin Resistance.
▼ Maintain lean body weight.
▼ Repair and maintain cell membranes.
▼ Balance hormones and improve hormone function.
▼ Improve blood glucose balance.
▼ Reduce inflammation in the body, by inhibiting inflammatory cytokines.
▼ Reduce the risk of death by heart attack by 30–50 percent.
▼ Control and even lower high cholesterol.
▼ Thin the blood and prevent high blood pressure, heart disease, strokes, and DVT (deep vein thrombosis).
▼ Resolve depression.
▼ Develop and maintain the nervous system including the eyes. Correcting deficiencies improves ADD, ADHD, dyslexia, and dyspraxia. Deficiencies are also found in Autistic Spectrum Disorders.

 Studies show that omega 3 fatty acids may help prevent heart disease and reduce incidence of sudden death from a heart attack by approximately 50 percent.*

Omega 6 family

Omega 6 essential fats help:

▼ Repair and maintain cell membranes, but to a lesser degree than omega 3.
▼ Lower cholesterol, again to a lesser degree than omega 3.
▼ Produce hormonelike compounds called prostaglandins, which can help reduce PMT (premenstrual tension) symptoms, dry skin for example.
▼ Improve blood glucose balance.
▼ Support the nervous system—deficiencies contribute to ADD, ADHD, dyslexia and dyspraxia, and are found in Autistic Spectrum Disorders.
▼ Reduce inflammation in the body.

---

* Albert et al., *NEJM*, 2002, 346, 1113–1118.

Omega 9 family

Omega 9 essential fats help:

▼ Protect against heart disease by reducing the oxidation (cell membrane damage) of LDL (bad) cholesterol.

The importance of vitamins and minerals

Certain enzymes play a key part in converting the essential fats into longer carbon chain fats and these enzymes require particular vitamins and minerals to exist. These are zinc, magnesium, biotin, vitamin C, vitamin B_6, and Vitamin B_3. Therefore, not only do we need to ensure that we eat the right kinds of fats but we also need to make sure we are eating foods rich in these key vitamins and minerals. It is extremely common to be deficient in one of these vitamins or minerals. (Chapter 8 will help you identify your vitamin and mineral deficiencies.)

Bad fats

Yes, there are definitely some fats that are bad for your health. However, it is usually a question of only eating them in moderation rather than cutting them out completely. The fats we're talking about are called saturated fats, which are in found in high quantities in animal products such as cheese, butter, and red meats. There are also some plant foods high in saturated fats, such as coconut and avocado, but these are better for you than their animal counterparts. As I mentioned in the last chapter, it is recommended that you limit your red meat intake to one or two meals a week. In the case of the vegetable saturated fats, you should also limit them to two or three. There is also a surprising benefit to coconut fats which we'll look at later.

The reason saturated fats can be bad for your health when eaten in excess is that they have been associated with heart disease and Insulin Resistance. They may contribute to raising blood fats, which encourages furring of the arteries and potentially heart attacks and strokes, quite apart from increasing body fat, itself a major risk for heart disease. The more overweight you are the fewer saturated fats you should eat.

Ugly fats

The really bad fats are called "trans" fats. These are the fats you really should avoid—of that there is no question. They are downright bad for your health and you shouldn't eat any at all. Unfortunately, they are almost exclusively used in processed foods to maintain their shelf life, and as a result you can quite easily eat them without being aware. Trans fats are produced by a manmade process, and never in nature. As a good guide, the longer the shelf life of a processed food that contains fat, the more likely it is that the fat is trans fat.

Trans fats are so bad for you because they block the function of essential fats, raise blood fats, and are strongly associated with heart disease. It's emerging that trans fats are now being linked with certain cancers. Perhaps worst of all for people with Insulin Resistance, trans fats actively disrupt insulin receptors, so the body releases more insulin to compensate. It is at the core of what goes wrong in Insulin Resistance. To emphasize how bad they are for you, it is even more important that you don't eat foods containing trans fats than it is for you to avoid foods containing refined sugar. That said, you'll often find foods containing trans fats contain sugar as well (e.g. cookies).

Know your trans fats

Trans fats are hidden in our food, labeled under various aliases
Partially hydrogenated vegetable oil or fat
Hydrogenated vegetable oil or fat
Simply as "vegetable oil" in processed foods
Even "pure vegetable oil" can contain trans fats

Getting the correct balance of essential fatty acids

Your body needs different quantities of the omega 3 and omega 6 fatty acids. Throughout our evolution the balance of omega 6 to omega 3 was about 1:1.* However, the modern diet contains a drastically different balance of omega 6 to omega 3 fats, and it is now more like

---

* S.C. Cunnance, L.S. Harbige and M.A. Crawford, 'The importance of energy and nutrient supply in human brain evolution,' *Nutr. Health,* 1993, 9, 219–235.

15–45:1. The main reason is the abundance of vegetable oils, such as corn, sunflower, soy, and cottonseed oils, in modern Western diets. This imbalance is certainly not benign and indirectly contributes to Insulin Resistance, as well as inflammatory and degenerative conditions such as arthritis. This is because the omega 6 pathways can convert to arachidonic acid, an inflammatory prostaglandin, as well as its anti-inflammatory prostaglandin (see diagram below). Omega 3 fatty acids, on the other hand, convert only to anti-inflammatory prostaglandins. A prostaglandin is a local hormonelike substance that influences inflammation in the body. If you have high levels of insulin this creates a pro-inflammatory environment in your body due to increased levels of arachidonic acid (see diagram below), derived from the omega 6 family fats. This in turn results in the production of more inflammatory cytokines (see chapter 4), which in turn increases Insulin Resistance. Thus, it may be necessary to supplement the diet with omega 3 fish oils, including EPA and DHA (e.g. Super EPA), in order to achieve maximum improvement of insulin sensitivity.

Insulin Resistance and fat metabolism

How hyperinsulinism effects EFA metabolism

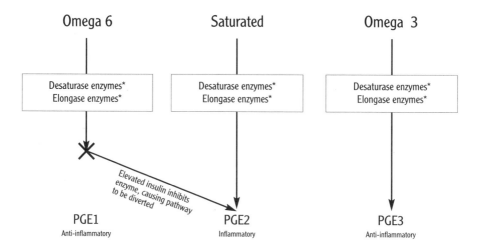

Omega 6	Saturated	Omega 3
Desaturase enzymes* Elongase enzymes*	Desaturase enzymes* Elongase enzymes*	Desaturase enzymes* Elongase enzymes*

Elevated insulin inhibits enzyme, causing pathway to be diverted

PGE1	PGE2	PGE3
Anti-inflammatory	Inflammatory	Anti-inflammatory

* Require cofactor nutrients: Zinc, Magnesium, Biotin, Vitamins C, B_3, B_6

If you are vegetarian with Insulin Resistance, you should note that the conversion of Alpha Linolenic Acid (ALA) (omega 3) to EPA and DHA is extremely poor, and simply consuming ALA is no guarantee that you will have enough EPA or DHA. If your views permit, it is highly recommended that you take a fish oil supplement that contains the preformed EPA and DHA, such as Super EPA (see chapter 14).

Low fat diets are bad for your health

If low fat diets really worked then there would be millions of slimmer, happier people around. The media and food industry have given fat such a bad name that people are terrified to eat it, thinking they will put on weight. Ironically, they turn to carbohydrate foods to replace the fats, which, as we discussed in chapter 2, is precisely what actually makes their weight problem worse. If you've got Insulin Resistance, and want to lose weight, you've got to make friends with the right fats, and ignore any media gossip—and that includes celebrity diets—promoting a fat-free existence. Foods that boast being virtually or totally fat free have normally had carbohydrates (e.g. sugar) added to compensate for both taste and texture. What this means is that the so-called "healthy option" foods that have reduced fat are actually less insulin-friendly than if they hadn't been tampered with at all. So next time you are out shopping, rather than looking for low fat look for sugarfree.

As further confirmation that low fat diets do not work, Walter Willett, MD, an eminent researcher at Harvard University, found that none of the low-fat weight-loss trials carried out over the past decade helped the participants lose weight.

So which oils should I eat?

The best oils are unrefined and mechanically pressed (expeller), or cold-pressed, without the use of harmful solvents. The oils should be as unaffected by the process as possible and that includes the taste, which should be like the nut or seed. The oils need to be stored in black or opaque containers that protect them from light, and they must be kept in a cool or cold place, which includes during shipping and storage. The containers must be airtight because oxygen is one of the three spoiling factors for these good oils. Once you have bought your oil, I suggest putting one of those special tops in the bottle that are used for wine bottles once they have been opened. This can minimize the exposure to air and oxygen that might otherwise affect the oil.

One of the most common misapprehensions about vegetable oils (e.g. corn and sunflower) is that they are the healthy ones when it comes to getting the right fats. All too often the ones on sale in the shops are not cold-pressed, not stored in dark containers and, even worse, are shelved under bright artificial lighting—you also have no idea about how they were shipped and stored. Although you should limit your intake of saturated fats, it's simply not true that these vegetable oils are better for you than saturated animal fats. This is particularly true if the vegetable oil has gone rancid, because it is then more harmful, particularly if you fry food with it.

To be fair, sesame oil is an exception because it is relatively stable due to its content of naturally occurring preservatives called sesamol and sesamin. Nonetheless, as with all oils, you should not expose it to high temperatures for more than a very short time.

Corn oil is usually solvent-extracted, and not recommended.

Olive oil is more stable than the above vegetable oils, but still should be used in its raw state and not fried with. If you have to fry food use butter or coconut fat.

Cooking and eating oils

Ideally, do not cook with an oil or fat. The heat transforms the fat into something that is damaged and damaging to your health. These damaged fats certainly contribute to Insulin Resistance, as well as to conditions such as heart disease.

Choose to broil, grill, steam, or bake instead of frying. Try frying with a small amount of water instead of oil. This is important for two reasons: one, you will not be using a fragile oil; and two, you will better preserve the nutritional status of what you are cooking.

To maintain the life of your oils store them in the fridge, including olive oil. It also helps if you add a few drops of the vitamin E liquid, called Bio E-Mulsion Forte, because this acts as an antioxidant, preventing it from turning rancid. If you use only modest amounts of oils, buy small bottles so they are not sitting around for long periods of time. Do use raw oils as dressings to pour over salads and vegetables, but always return them to the fridge and airtight containers.

Oils that you can cook with

Butter, coconut fat, and palm oil are the safest to cook with because they are high in the stable, saturated fats which are much less affected by heat and air, and contain virtually no unstable unsaturated fats.

How much and how often should I eat essential fats?

Aim to eat oily fish two to four times a week, and do add olive oil to your food everyday, as desired. Also eat fresh, dark green vegetables raw or cooked every day. Vegetarians should eat a portion of fresh nuts (not peanuts or pine kernels) or seeds daily, such as walnuts, pumpkin seeds, or sunflower seeds. A portion is about a ¼–½ a cup. If you are vegetarian, you will almost certainly need to take a supplement containing omega 3 fats such, as linseed oil.

So what supplements should I take?

If you scored 4 or more in the Fats Questionnaire you are likely to be deficient in omega 3 fats and probably deficient in good-quality omega 6 fats. To correct this as quickly as possible, you should take supplements as directed by the Good Fat Supplement Plan in chapter 14.

If you scored 10 or more and your BMI is over 25, you should also take additional Carnitine, an amino acid that not only improves insulin sensitivity but also improves the metabolism of fats.

A note on purity

There are different qualities of fish oils and it is important to purchase a high-quality product. This is because poorer grade fish oils can contain heavy metals, such as mercury, and other toxins. Molecular distillation is the best processing method for fish oil supplements, so check before you buy. Usually price reflects quality (i.e. the cheapest fish oils may well not be the purest). Good-quality fish oil supplements are recommended in chapter 14.

Summary of key points

▼ The right fats are essential for your health and help reverse Insulin Resistance.

▼ The unsaturated essential fats omega 6 and, particularly, omega 3 are the most important fats. Aim to eat them every day.

▼ Limit your intake of saturated animal fats to one or two times a week and, if you eat them, limit your intake of saturated vegetable fats to two or three times.

▼ Trans fats are extremely bad for your health and directly contribute to Insulin Resistance and heart disease. They should be strictly avoided.

▼ Most processed and packaged foods that have any fat in them contain trans fats.

▼ If you must fry anything, the only fats you should use are butter, coconut butter, and palm oil. All other unsaturated fats, including olive oil and sunflower oil, are damaged when heated and in turn are damaging to your health.

▼ Eat unsaturated oils raw by pouring them over salads or vegetables.

▼ Take a fish oil supplement to help you consume optimum amounts of omega 3 fat.

7 Antioxidants: Your Defense Against Excess Insulin

The Insulin Connection

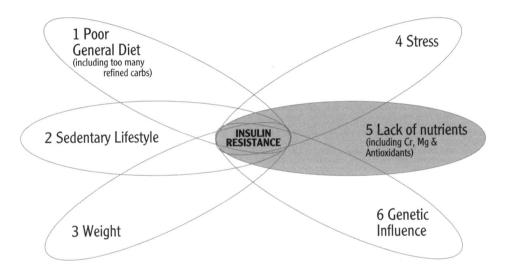

There is a lot of talk in the media about the wonders of antioxidants and how they help prevent disease and premature aging. This is certainly true and they also protect you from Insulin Resistance. As the name suggests, antioxidants basically defend the body from oxidative stress, which damages cell membranes. We will look at this in more detail later. Certain antioxidants are particularly useful in helping you to reverse Insulin Resistance and this chapter explains what they are and which foods and supplements provide them. Let's begin, however, with a questionnaire to see if you are getting enough antioxidants.

The Antioxidant Questionnaire

This is the longest questionnaire in the book, which tells you that there are many potential factors that increase your need for antioxidants. If you score highly, then you'll be pleased to know that you can usually improve your antioxidant reserves quickly.

Scoring the questionnaire

Answer "yes" or "no" to the following questions. Each "yes" answer is given a single point.

Do you:

1 Smoke cigarettes every day?
2 Smoke more than 10 cigarettes a day on average?
3 Take any other drugs regularly (prescription or recreational)?
4 Live or work in a smoky environment?
5 Drink more than 2 glasses of alcohol a day?
6 Binge drink more than twice a month (e.g. more than 4 drinks at a time)?
7 Eat refined sugar every day?
8 Eat refined sugar every four days or less?
9 Eat refined sugar once or twice a week?
10 Eat fewer than three servings of vegetables a day?
11 Eat less than one serving of vegetables a day?
12 Eat fewer than two pieces of fruit a day?
13 Eat fewer than 5 pieces of fruit a week?
14 Live in a city?
15 Walk or exercise by busy roads?
16 Work in or around a lot of electrical equipment (e.g. computers)?
17 Eat fried food every week?
18 Eat burned or blackened food every week?
19 Eat trans or processed fats (typically found in processed foods, including oatmeal bars, preprepared meals, etc.)?
20 Exercise intensively every week?
21 Exercise for more than two hours more than twice a week?
22 Have a BMI greater than 25?

23 Have a BMI greater than 30?

24 Get low blood sugar symptoms (hypoglycemia)?

25 Get sugar cravings?

26 Regularly miss meals?

27 Get anxious and stressed every week?

28 Get anxious and stressed every day?

29 Rush from task to task most of the time?

30 Do a job that involves performing (e.g. acting, giving speeches, or presentations)?

31 Have disturbed sleep or insomnia?

32 Bruise easily?

33 Have a family history of cancer or diabetes or heart disease?

34 Have cataracts?

35 Have diabetes (type I or II)?

36 Have Insulin Resistance?

Total score =   /36

Interpreting the questionnaire

0–6   Well done, your lifestyle and diet does not appear to be a major source of oxidative stress. This is good if you have any degree of Insulin Resistance. However, if you smoke, try to cut down or ideally give up. Right now, though, you'll need to increase your intake of antioxidants from your food. If you are following one of the Insulin Resistance Supplement Plans you won't need to add any other specific antioxidant supplements, because they already contain a significant number of antioxidants.

7–16 You would benefit from increasing your antioxidant intake. Start implementing the Insulin Factor Diet Plan, and think about what steps you could take to reduce lifestyle and environmental stresses in your life. Oxidative stress could well be a contributory factor to your Insulin Resistance. In addition to whatever Insulin Resistance Supplement Plan you are following, follow the Antioxidant Supplement Plan A. Please redo this questionnaire in four weeks' time to see if you need to continue with it.

17–24 There is a strong need for you to increase your antioxidant intake. You really should start to follow the Insulin Factor Diet Plan, consider taking necessary steps to reduce stress (see chapter 9), and change any controllable aspects of your environment. Oxidative stress is strongly indicated as a contributory factor to your Insulin Resistance. In addition to whatever Insulin Resistance Supplement Plan you are following, follow the Antioxidant Supplement Plan B. Please redo this questionnaire in four weeks' time to see if you can reduce to Plan A.

25+ You have an immediate and strong need to boost your antioxidant intake. At the same time, you really should begin to change your diet by following the Insulin Factor Diet Plan, take steps to reduce stress (see chapter 9) and aspects of your environment. Oxidative stress is almost certainly contributing to your Insulin Resistance. Every aspect of your health should benefit from taking both the Insulin Resistance Supplement Plan as well as the Antioxidant Supplement Plan C. Please redo this questionnaire in four weeks' time to see if you can reduce to Plan B.

What is oxidative stress?

Oxidative stress is a natural phenomenon in any creature that breathes oxygen, so we're designed to be able to cope with it. Oxidative stress is also called free radical damage, and involves unstable oxygen molecules, "free radicals," which can damage cells in our bodies. Antioxidants in the body counter oxidative stress, and oxidative stress will only become a problem when it is greater than the body's antioxidant reserves. When this happens it causes a domino effect of cell damage in the body. Over time, this can ultimately result in overt signs and symptoms of disease, such as heart disease, arthritis, and cancers. One of the most credible theories on aging centers on oxidative stress—the more oxidative stress you have, the quicker you age.

The Insulin Factor Plan is effectively an antiaging plan

When you reverse Insulin Resistance, at the same you will also be rejuvenating your metabolism. A healthy metabolism is the key to being healthy in every way—you look and feel good. Not only will you be less susceptible to illness, but your skin will look glowing (it won't show signs of premature aging), you'll be leaner and more toned, and you will drastically cut your chances of getting any degenerative diseases. In short, you will increase your lifespan and improve your quality of life.

Oxidative stress is caused by both internal metabolism and external factors, such as pollution of all kinds including fumes from traffic exhaust fumes and office machinery, toxic chemicals, exposure to heavy metals (i.e. mercury and lead) or radiation, and electromagnetic exposure (e.g. X-rays), passive or active smoking, and so on. Eating food that has been browned or burned, particularly on a barbeque, also causes oxidative stress. It may shock you to know that a large barbequed meal causes as much oxidative stress as smoking an entire pack of cigarettes. Oxidative stress is now more of a problem because not only have sources of oxidative stress increased but we tend to eat fewer antioxidants in our diet.

Antioxidants and Insulin Resistance

Oxidative stress also damages insulin receptor cells and contributes to Insulin Resistance. Evidence now shows that people who have weight problems are actually manifesting signs of oxidative stress damage. This is because insulin receptor cells have already been damaged and insulin is becoming less efficient.

The more insulin cell receptors are damaged the more oxidative stress is caused. This is because the less efficient your body becomes at storing blood glucose and the higher the insulin level, the more oxidative stress and free radicals are produced. This becomes a vicious cycle and, in order to break it, you need to dramatically increase your antioxidant intake. Once you do, the inflammatory immune messengers called cytokines (see chapter 4) will also be tempered, further helping to reduce Insulin Resistance. Perhaps not surprisingly, specific nutrients that have been found to improve insulin sensitivity do so at least in part due to their antioxidant effect.

Foods and antioxidants

Your primary source of antioxidants should be the food you eat every day. Natural foods contain a wide array of substances that offer antioxidant benefits. These start to diminish the moment they are picked or harvested, which is why it is always better to eat food that is as fresh as possible. Virtually every food from strawberries to spinach and carrots contain beneficial antioxidants. The following foods are rich sources of various plant antioxidants and should form a major part of your diet. These are included in the Insulin Factor Diet Plan.

Selected foods rich in plant antioxidants

Food	Name of important antioxidant
Acerola cherries, guavas, red peppers, kale, broccoli	vitamin C
Avocado, asparagus, watermelon	glutathione
Berries, red grapes, red wine	polyphenols, flavonoids
Blackcurrants, cranberries, raspberries	anthocyanidins
Broccoli	indole-3-carbinol (I3C), diindolylmethane (DIM)
Cabbage, Brussels sprouts	sulforapohanes
Carrots	beta carotene
Citrus fruit (oranges, lemons)	vitamin C, limonenes
Cranberries	anthocyanidins
Garlic	allicin
Green leafy vegetables	magnesium, lutein, chlorophyll
Linseed (flax)	lignans
Onions, parsley	4-oxo-flavonoids
Orange vegetables & fruit	alpha-carotene
Peaches	bioflavans
Soy	isoflavones: genistein, daidzein, saponins, phytosterols
Strawberries, tea, red wine	catechins
Tomatoes	lycopene, coumarins

The greater the degree of Insulin Resistance you have and the higher your scores in the Insulin Resistance Questionnaire and the Antioxidant Questionnaire, the more of these foods you should eat. It is very difficult to eat enough antioxidants anyway, but if you have any degree of Insulin Resistance it is harder still. For this reason, you will need to follow one of the Antioxidant Supplement Plans in chapter 14. Your Antioxidant Questionnaire score will determine which of the three plans you should follow.

Summary of key points

▼ Antioxidants are necessary for everyone because they protect against aging and degenerative disease.
▼ The modern diet is low in antioxidants.
▼ Oxidative stress is more prevalent today than ever before.
▼ Antioxidants play a key role in protecting cell membranes from damage that directly leads to Insulin Resistance.
▼ Colorful plant foods are a rich source of antioxidants and should be eaten every day.
▼ When you have Insulin Resistance you need to take antioxidant supplements.

8 Key Nutrients to Reverse Insulin Resistance

The Insulin Connection

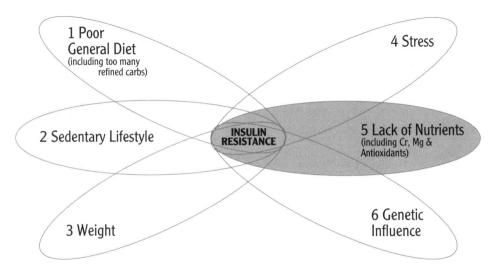

1 Poor General Diet (including too many refined carbs)

2 Sedentary Lifestyle

3 Weight

INSULIN RESISTANCE

4 Stress

5 Lack of Nutrients (including Cr, Mg & Antioxidants)

6 Genetic Influence

This chapter focuses on the role of specific vitamins, minerals, and plant extracts that will help you reverse Insulin Resistance. It will also help you understand why certain nutrients are so important in helping you reverse Insulin Resistance, which foods are good sources of these, and why you should include them in your diet. As you will see in chapter 13, many of these foods are included in the basic recipes and meal plans to get you started.

One of the six major causes of Insulin Resistance is a lack of vital nutrients, including vitamins and minerals. When you don't eat enough of these or you eat too many refined, processed foods it makes it harder for insulin to do its job as efficiently. Obviously, in your diet, you should be aiming to get an overall balance of vitamins and minerals, but when you are insulin resistant, there are five key minerals and three vital vitamins that you need to focus on. The good news is that if you eat the foods rich in these nutrients, you will also be getting a good balance of all the other remaining essential vitamins and minerals.

Key minerals and vitamins to reverse Insulin Resistance

Minerals

Chromium

Magnesium

Zinc

Vanadium

Calcium

Vitamins

Vitamin B_6 (pyridoxine)

Vitamin B_3 (niacin/nacinamide)

Biotin

Vitamins and minerals work best as a team

With vitamins and minerals, it is not just a question of eating or taking supplements of one or two but about getting a balance. This is because they work synergistically, i.e. they depend on each other to be able to work best in the body. For this reason, it is NOT recommended that you take one nutrient by itself without a good balance of others. In aid of this, the Insulin Resistance Supplement Plans contain a wide range of nutrients, including the most important vitamins and minerals described in this chapter. The Insulin Factor Diet Plan will help you choose foods rich in these nutrients, and the Insulin Resistance Questionnaire in chapter 3 will direct you to the appropriate Supplement Plan in chapter 14.

Chromium

Chromium is well known for its role in helping to balance blood sugar levels and control insulin levels. Chromium supplementation alone has been shown to help reduce body weight, increase lean muscle, and even decrease high levels of cholesterol and blood fats. Each of the three Insulin Resistance Supplement Plans do include chromium in the recommended Glucobalance formula, but it is still important that you eat as many foods as you can that are high in this nutrient.

 Chromium is one of the most important nutrients for reversing Insulin Resistance; it is also the nutrient depleted most by refining and processing food.

Unfortunately, if you eat a diet high in refined carbohydrates, grains, and sugars, you will deplete your intake of chromium by as much as 97 percent. Furthermore this type of diet increases the excretion of chromium from your body by as much as 300 percent.*

Chromium, exercise, and insulin

You don't just need to look at your diet when it comes to maintaining your chromium levels. If you lead a sedentary lifestyle, not only will your insulin levels be higher and therefore your need for chromium be higher, but your body will also be losing more chromium than it would if you exercised moderately. This is because a certain amount of muscle activity helps the body retain chromium.

---

* A.S. Kozlovsky, P.B. Moser, S. Reiser and R.A. Anderson, 'Effects of diets high in simple sugars on chromium urinary losses,' *Metabolism*, 1986, 35, 515–518; R.A. Anderson, N.A. Bryden, M.M. Polansky and S. Reiser, 'Urinary chromium excretion and insulinogenic properties of carbohydrates,' *Am. J. Clin. Nutr.*, 1990, 1, 864–868

Good sources of chromium

Peanuts	Wheat germ	Parsnips
Brewer's yeast	Green string beans	Lamb
Prunes	Spinach	Scallops
Calves' liver	Broccoli	Celery (raw)
Clams	Green bell peppers	Banana
Whole-wheat bread	Onions	Beef
Wheat bran	Dark green lettuce	Oysters
Peas	Pears	Carrots
Corn	Cabbage	Lentils
Rye bread	Potatoes	Navy beans
Chicken breast	Watercress	Leeks
Mushrooms (raw)	Brussels sprouts	Eggs
Tomatoes (raw)	Apples	

A Note on yeast

Unfortunately, many people should not eat too much yeast because they have problems with candida, a yeast that lives within the digestive tract. If you have a yeast sensitivity, choose other chromium-rich foods.

Can chromium be toxic?

If you saw the movie *Erin Brockovich* you might remember that it focused on a community that had been poisoned by chromium. Rest assured, it was NOT the form of chromium you find in food or supplements. It was the toxic form of chromium, the hexavalent type (IV).

Magnesium

Magnesium deficiency is as common as a deficiency in chromium. Like chromium, the process of refining foods destroys much of its magnesium content. Similarly, it is not just a question of diet, but of other factors too, such as stress, which deplete magnesium from your body.

Magnesium has numerous biological functions, not least in the way it supports insulin function. It is also one of the most important nutrients for energy, and fatigue is one of the first signs of magnesium deficiency. Magnesium is also involved in fat metabolism.

Magnesium and mood

Interestingly, there is a link between magnesium deficiency and poor mood and depression. This is because magnesium is your body's calming mineral, and is needed to help produce serotonin, the "antidepressant" brain chemical. If you are continually stressed, your body uses up magnesium much more quickly, diverting it from its other functions including serotonin metabolism. See chapter 9 for more about stress.

Magnesium and oxidative stress

There is a very real link between magnesium and oxidative stress, or free radical damage (see chapter 7). This is because oxidative stress doesn't just damage insulin cell receptors, but also damages the cell receptors that are involved in absorbing magnesium. Therefore, if you are not getting enough antioxidants to counter oxidative stress, you are likely to be magnesium deficient. This would also make you feel more tired and depressed.

Good sources of magnesium

Rich sources	Good sources
Kelp	Soybeans
Wheat germ	Brown rice
Almonds	Figs (dried)
Cashews	Avocado
Molasses, blackstrap	Parsley
Brewer's yeast	Sunflower seeds
Buckwheat	Barley
Brazil nuts	Garlic
Hazelnuts	Peas
Peanuts	Banana
Millet	Sweet potato
Wheat grain	Broccoli
Pecan	Cauliflower
Walnuts	Carrot
Rye	Celery
Tofu	Milk

Like chromium, you will need to supplement your diet with magnesium so this is included in the Insulin Resistance Supplement Plans in chapter 14.

Zinc

Zinc is a key mineral with regard to insulin function because it is necessary for the synthesis of insulin and the way it helps insulin bind to cell receptors. It will come as no surprise that zinc deficiency is extremely common, particularly among people who are insulin resistant. Zinc is also essential for stomach acid production, which is needed for the proper digestion of food and absorption of all nutrients. If you are zinc deficient this affects the amount of stomach acid you can produce so you become less effective at digesting foods. This is a vicious cycle because the less stomach acid you have the lower the level of zinc. If your diet is high in refined foods, your levels of zinc will already be low.

Good sources of zinc

Oysters	Brazil nuts	Hazelnuts
Wheat germ	Milk	Muesli
Sesame seeds	Liver	Shrimp
Pumpkin seeds	Peanuts	Macadamia nuts
Cashews	Turkey	Soy beans
Crab	Lobster	Chickpeas
Beef/veal	Almonds	Baked beans
Pecans	Chicken	
Sunflower seeds	Walnuts	
Lamb	Whole-wheat bread	

Like chromium and magnesium, you will need to supplement your diet with zinc so this is included in the Insulin Resistance Supplement Plans in chapter 14.

Vanadium

Vanadium is a little-known trace mineral that behaves like chromium and improves insulin function. Vanadium can be as important as chromium in balancing blood glucose levels.

Good sources of vanadium

Buckwheat	Olive oil	Onions
Parsley	Sunflower seeds	Whole-wheat bread
Soybeans	Green string beans	Apples
Safflower oil	Carrots	Dark green lettuce
Sunflower oil	Garlic	
Oats	Tomatoes	

Like the other minerals, you will need to supplement your diet with vanadium so this is included in the Insulin Resistance Supplement Plans in chapter 14.

Calcium

New research indicates that calcium is a more important mineral than previously recognized in reversing Insulin Resistance. A lack of calcium can upset the proper flow of nutrients into your cells, and influences how well insulin works. About 50 percent of women and 25 percent of men are estimated to consume less than the RDI (Recommended Daily Intake) for calcium,* making calcium deficiency another contributory factor in the rising incidence of Insulin Resistance.

---

* Technical Catalog 2002–2003, Lamberts Healthcare Ltd.

Calcium and fat loss

Calcium has increasingly been shown to be strongly associated with fat metabolism. In one study, women on high calcium diets lost weight more easily than similar women on similar calorie diets.* In another study, Doctors Michael and Paula Zemel found that by simply adding yogurt to the diet of a group of obese people, they lost 11 pounds of fat in a year, compared to a group who did not eat yogurt. This is partly explained by an enzyme called fatty acid synthase, which stimulates the storing of fat, and was found to be about 2.5 times higher with a low calcium diet. However, the levels of this enzyme decrease when you increase the amount of calcium you eat. It can also be explained by the fact that a high calcium diet increases your body's ability to burn fat by as much as 300–500 percent.

Calcium and cravings

Calcium not only helps to burn excess fat, it also helps reduce food cravings. Calcium has a "buffering" effect, in that it helps neutralize excess acid in your body. When combined with certain other nutrients, this buffering effect can eliminate or reduce cravings of many different kinds. Calcium also helps improve the feeling of being satisfied after eating.

In one particularly interesting study, patients who were seriously addicted to stimulant drugs and alcohol found their withdrawal symptoms reduced by 90 percent when they were given a combination of calcium and vitamin C.

Dietary sources of calcium

There is a lot of controversy surrounding good sources of calcium, particularly when it comes to dairy products. Contrary to popular belief, milk is not the wonder source of calcium that it is made out to be. Up until the age of about 18, when children and teenagers are still growing, milk is certainly a helpful source of calcium, when

---

* C.M. Weaver, R. Heaney, M. Shils et al., eds, *Modern Nutrition in Health and Disease*, 9th edition, 1999, Lippincott, Williams and Wilkins, pp. 141–143.

other rich sources of calcium are less likely to be consumed. However, in adults, milk should be consumed sparingly (less than two pints a week), because a higher consumption can cause a relative deficiency of magnesium. You may think that drinking more milk helps protect you from arthritis and osteoporosis when, in fact, the opposite is true. The highest rates of osteoporosis occur in the countries that drink the most milk. One prime reason for this is the fact that the protein in milk acidifies the blood, and the body uses calcium from bone to buffer it. The net effect can be bone loss. Milk fat (animal fat) contributes to inflammation in the body, and for this reason may also contribute to arthritis. In addition, milk and cheese products are one of the most common sources of food intolerance, which can readily contribute to both arthritis and cause gut inflammation which increases your risk of Insulin Resistance. (Yogurt, especially natural live yogurt, is much easier to digest so it's fine to eat it regularly.) So, rather than drink lots of milk and eat cheese every day, choose other calcium-rich foods from the list below.

Good sources of calcium

Sesame seeds (& tahini)	Shrimp
Sardines	Black beans
Tofu/ Tempeh	Pinto beans
Collard greens	Salmon
Spinach (raw)	Almonds

In the USA, the RDI (Recommended Daily Intake) for calcium is 1,000mg, but it varies in other countries, highlighting the uncertainty of ideal levels. While this can be achieved by dietary means, it is not recommended for the reasons above that you do so with dairy products alone—natural, live yogurt is the most healthy dairy source of calcium. However, many people need supplements to make sure they're getting enough calcium. This is particularly true if you avoid dairy products completely or if you are insulin resistant, or find it difficult to eat the alternatives.

As with the four other key minerals, you will need to supplement your diet with calcium so this is included in the Insulin Resistance Supplement Plans in chapter 14. Additional calcium in the form of Calcium Magnesium Citrate is also recommended in the Supplement Plans.

Vitamin B_6

Vitamin B_6, or pyridoxine, is a cofactor in hundreds of different reactions in the human body. Among its many roles, vitamin B_6 supports hormonal balance and when deficient it can cause blood glucose problems. In fact, in the opinion of certain clinicians, a vitamin B_6 deficiency causes diabetes and gestational diabetes.

As with minerals, refined, processed foods are depleted in vitamin B_6. In addition, there are also an increasing number of dietary and lifestyle factors that prevent vitamin B_6 from being absorbed or used properly in the body or hasten its excretion. This includes food colorings (FD&C yellow No.5), the contraceptive pill, alcohol, and some prescription drugs.

Good sources of vitamin B_6 (pyridoxine)

Wholegrain cereals	Buckwheat flour	Avocado
Muesli	Walnuts	Lamb
Sunflower seeds	Turkey	Potato
Wheat germ	Pork & ham	Prunes
Liver	Kidney beans	Cashews
Sesame seeds	Seaweed (spirulina)	Brazil nuts
Hazelnuts	Whole-wheat bread	Haricot beans
Lentils	Tuna	Soymilk
Chicken	Kale	
Bananas	Peanuts	

You will need to supplement your diet with vitamin B_6 so this is included in the Insulin Resistance Supplement Plans in chapter 14.

Vitamin B_3 (niacin)

Vitamin B_3 is also of critical importance to Insulin Resistance because it works with chromium to help balance blood glucose. As with all other nutrients, the refining and processing of foods reduces dietary content of vitamin B_3, and at the same time increases the need for it.

Good sources of niacin

Wholegrain cereals	Mackerel	Sunflower seeds
Liver	Venison	Peaches
Peanuts	Lamb	Black beans
Chicken	Pork & ham	Whole-wheat bread
Seaweed (spirulina)	Rice flour	Mushrooms
Rabbit	Wheat germ	Herring
Tuna	Turkey	Brown rice
Puffed wheat	Sardines	Navy beans
Salmon	Duck	
Halibut	Sesame seeds	

You will also need to supplement your diet with vitamin B_3 so this is included in the Insulin Resistance Supplement Plans in chapter 14.

Biotin

Biotin is also known as vitamin H. It is involved in the metabolism of fats, carbohydrates, and proteins. Your body needs biotin to metabolize carbohydrate into glucose and control blood glucose levels. Interestingly, higher levels of biotin can have a similar effect to chromium and lower elevated blood glucose, which is of vital importance if you have Insulin Resistance.

Good sources of biotin

Liver	Oysters	Salmon
Walnuts	Peas	Raisins
Peanuts	Puffed wheat cereal	Tomato
Almonds	Spinach (raw)	Watermelon
Eggs	Sardines	Cherries
Cauliflower	Crab	Bananas
Lentils	Halibut	Sweet potato
Herring	Whole-wheat bread	
Lima beans	Haddock	

As with vitamins B_6 and B_3, you will need to supplement your diet with biotin so this is included in the Insulin Resistance Supplement Plans in chapter 14.

Powerful help from nature

In addition to the eight key vitamins and minerals there are also some remarkably effective plant extracts that can help to optimize blood glucose and minimize insulin levels. Three of the most potent known are:

1 Alpha lipoic acid
2 Corosolic acid
3 Silymarin (Milk Thistle extract)

Alpha lipoic acid

Alpha lipoic acid, known simply as lipoic acid, is an antioxidant found in broccoli, spinach, and other dark green leafy vegetables. It has a number of special properties but it is not termed an "essential" nutrient, because small amounts of it can be made in the body. However, the amount the body makes is neglible if you eat a diet high in refined carbohydrates, are overweight, lead a sedentary lifestyle, and suffer from stress. To make matters worse, levels of lipoic acid naturally decrease with age and are associated with less efficient blood glucose control.

Lipoic acid possesses an ability to lower insulin and blood glucose levels and restore the body's ability to burn glucose efficiently. This, combined with its potent antioxidant properties, makes it one of the most important nutrients for anyone with Insulin Resistance. Since its recent arrival on the nutrition scene, we've been using lipoic acid with great effect at The Nutrition Clinic. Because it lowers a high glucose and insulin to normal, lipoic acid removes the prime causes of oxidative stress (see chapter 7) and therefore reduces inflammation and cell damage.

Lipoic acid is not only a potent antioxidant in its own right (it is both water and fat soluble) but it also recycles other antioxidants in your body (vitamins C and E, CoEnzyme Q10 and Glutathione), thereby increasing their active "shelf life" in the body.

How does it work?

Lipoic acid functions in the energy factories of our cells—the mitochondria. Mitochondria are engaged in effectively trapping energy and releasing it in a controlled manner for our body to use. However, mitochondria are exposed to free radicals and, because they lack DNA repair enzymes, they are therefore very reliant on antioxidant enzymes such as lipoic acid and coenzyme Q10. Lipoic acid serves to protect the oxygen-rich energy process and reduces the potential for free radical formation.* In this way it

---

* T. Konrad, P. Vivina, K. Kusterer et al., 'A-lipoic acid treatment decreases serum lactate and pyruvate concentrations and improves glucose effectiveness in lean and obese patients with type 2 diabetes,' *Diabetes Care*, 1999, 22: 280–287.

helps our bodies use glucose more effectively, a particularly key function when Insulin Resistance exists.

Lipoic acid improves the rate at which mitochondria can use glucose for energy by as much as twice the usual rate. When glucose is being burned up more quickly, and there is less risk of oxidative stress thanks to the antioxidant effects, it means that less glucose will be in the bloodstream and less insulin will be needed.* In this way, lipoic acid has rejuvenating effects on the major aspect of human metabolism.

The Insulin Resistance Supplement Plans in chapter 14 include Lipoic Acid.

Corosolic acid

Corosolic acid is derived from the tropical botanical plant called *Lagerstroemia speciosa L.*, also known as Queen's flower, Pride of India, or Banaba. The leaf tea or extract has been used for centuries in Asia as an aid for blood sugar control, as well as for weight loss. Corosolic acid can be found in a supplement called GlucoFit™, which is a unique formulation containing the extract from these leaves.

It works by improving the transport of glucose into cells, thereby mimicking insulin's storage of glucose into cells. Human studies in Japan at the Tokyo Jikeikai Medical School have shown that while corosolic acid reduces high blood glucose levels, it does not lower a normal or low level of blood glucose. There is evidence to suggest that it even helps individuals who have low blood glucose by improving how their body uses glucose for energy. The participants taking corosolic acid had a beneficial "side effect" of weight loss. Furthermore, even a one-time dose had a lasting effect for several days. Studies show that the optimal dose of corosolic acid is 48mg per day in an oil-based soft gelatin capsule formulation, which you will get from two capsules of GlucoFit.

Because GlucoFit improves blood glucose and insulin levels, it reduces oxidative stress by default, and therefore has potent antioxi-

---

* S.K. Jain and G. Lim, 'Lipoic acid (LA) decreases protein glycation and increases (Na++K+) and Ca++-ATPases activities in high glucose (G)-treated red blood cells (RBC),' *Free Radical Biology & Medicine*, 1998, 25: S94, Abstract #268.

dant properties. GlucoFit is so effective an antioxidant that is has been compared to vitamin E.

Case Study: Mr. Andrews

This case history shows how beneficial GlucoFit can be if you are insulin resistant. Mr Andrews is a noninsulin-dependent diabetic, who had been overweight for most of his 65 years, usually weighing in at 210–223 pounds. However, having been diabetic for 3 years, his weight had increased to 258 pounds. Because he could not tolerate metformin (a commonly used drug for lowering blood sugar), because it caused him gastrointestinal distress, he was taking insulin and the latter had caused his weight gain. He sought advice from his doctor before implementing nutritional changes and, because he measured his glucose levels every day, he was confident that any changes could be compensated for. His existing diet was low in carbohydrates and free of all refined carbohydrates.

He had probably had a degree of Insulin Resistance for decades, so it was going to be a challenge to bring about a positive change. I prepared a complete nutritional and exercise program for him, which included the use of GlucoFit, lipoic acid, and Glucobalance. However, he only took GlucoFit to begin with in order not to "rock the boat" too much and alter the need for insulin too rapidly. In the very first week, however, before any change in exercise or diet had occurred, Mr. Andrews managed to reduce his insulin levels by 37 percent without altering his glucose level and lost 5 pounds in weight. These benefits were maintained over the first month when he lost 7 pounds, despite overeating, drinking alcohol on a number of occasions, and not changing his exercise habits. His blood glucose was 2 points lower than when he had taken 3 metformin per day together with insulin (before he had to stop the former), and was marginally elevated from the normal range.

So, he hadn't changed his exercise, he hadn't addressed his stress levels, but there had been a rapid and significant reduction in his insulin needs. This is a clear illustration of the effectiveness of GlucoFit.

Silymarin (Milk Thistle extract)

Milk Thistle is an herb that has long been used in traditional medicine, particularly for liver support. It contains a group of antioxidants, called silymarin, which are beneficial to a number of liver disorders. However, human trials with diabetics who also had liver disease have shown that it has a positive effect on blood glucose and insulin levels.

The benefits of the trial which lasted for a whole year were as follows:

1 Fasting insulin reduced by over 45 percent (increased insulin sensitivity)
2 Daily insulin requirements reduced by 23 percent
3 Fasting glucose reduced by 8.5 percent
4 Average daily glucose reduced by 14.8 percent
5 Silymarin group did not experience hypoglycemic episodes
6 Glucose levels in urine decreased by 40 percent
7 Oxidative stress marker reduced

The dose used in the above trial was 600mg of silymarin. A person with full-blown Insulin Resistance would probably need to take a lower dose. If you have digestive problems Milk Thistle extract will also help to reduce the resulting high levels of inflammatory cytokines (see chapter 4). How much silymarin you should take is detailed in the Insulin Resistance Supplement Plans in chapter 14.

There are a number of other traditional herbs that work in synergy with silymarin, and these include phyllanthus and dandelion. The three herb extracts have been combined in one synergistic formula called Phyllanthus Complex by Allergy Research Group. Each capsule provides 200mg of each of the standardized extracts.

Case Study: Mr. Patel

The case is an example of full-blown Insulin Resistance, bordering on diabetes. Mr. Patel was 50 years old, weighed 254 pounds and was 5 feet 10 inches tall. He also had many other chronic health imbalances relating to the gut and the liver. Neither GlucoFit nor lipoic acid were available at that time, but I recommended Glucobalance and Phyllanthus Complex (which includes silymarin) as part of his overall nutrition and exercise program.

Mr. Patel's initial fasting insulin level was 103 mIU/L, which is extremely high (the reference level is under 10 mIU/L). Having followed the program for about a month, he reported an initial weight loss of 9–11 pounds. Unfortunately, he had not been able to follow the dietary guidelines and had regained this weight as a consequence of overeating (this was one of the health problems). However, his next insulin result was 62 mIU/L. While this was still very high, it was 40 percent lower than it had been a month earlier—and this was in spite of no change in weight, exercise, or stress levels. Once again, this is an example of how potent a natural plant extract can be, without the side effects of drugs.

Summary of key points

▼ The key nutrients that will help reverse Insulin Resistance are the minerals chromium, magnesium, zinc, vanadium, and calcium, and the vitamins B_3, B_6, and biotin.

▼ In isolation, no single nutrient solves a metabolic problem on the scale of Insulin Resistance; a balanced combination of nutrients is most effective.

▼ Eat a varied diet of fresh, whole foods that contain a richer and wider variety of nutrients than a diet dominated by refined and processed food.

▼ Processed and refined foods actually deplete your nutrient intake and your body's ability to hold onto them.

▼ The swiftest way to reverse your Insulin Resistance is to follow the Insulin Factor Diet and Supplement Plans.

▼ Certain plant extracts can also have a potent effect on improving insulin and glucose levels, as well as improving antioxidant status, namely lipoic acid, GlucoFit and silymarin.

▼ These plant extracts can reduce need for medications.

▼ Used together with dietary changes, appropriate exercise, and stress reduction, the effects are likely to be additive.

Part Three

Could Your Lifestyle Be Contributing to Insulin Resistance?

9 Is Stress Affecting You More Than You Think?

The Insulin Connection

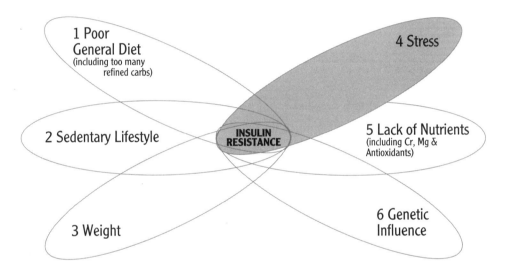

1 Poor General Diet (including too many refined carbs)

2 Sedentary Lifestyle

3 Weight

INSULIN RESISTANCE

4 Stress

5 Lack of Nutrients (including Cr, Mg & Antioxidants)

6 Genetic Influence

Stress is, of course, a natural part of life and the right amount of it is essential for our well-being. Unfortunately, with our hectic modern lifestyles, and diets high in refined carbohydrates, most of us have too much stress, as reflected by a recent survey. In *The New England Journal of Medicine*, it was reported that stress was markedly increased across the whole of the U.S. after the September 11 terrorist attacks. Forty-four percent of the adults questioned reported one or more substantial symptoms of stress; 90 percent had one or more symptoms to at least some degree. So, why is stress so relevant to Insulin Resistance? The answer is simple: because stress increases adrenal hormones and adrenal hormones increase Insulin Resistance. There is more to it than that, but that is it in a nutshell.

In this chapter we examine the stress response and the various factors that contribute to it. The adrenal stress questionnaire gives an indication of your status with regard to this vital factor in Insulin Resistance—and health in general—and how you can go about improving it. This is an integral part of the program to improve insulin sensitivity, and for some may be an underlying issue of even more importance than insulin.

Adrenal Stress Questionnaire

The two main adrenal hormones that have a direct influence on Insulin Resistance are cortisol and DHEA. Insulin Resistance is affected by these two hormones when cortisol is too high or too low, and DHEA is too low. Confusing as it may sound, many of the signs and symptoms that relate to high cortisol also mimic those of low cortisol (low cortisol production usually follows an extended period of high cortisol production). For some people, it is therefore not always straightforward to estimate the level of cortisol based on signs and symptoms. Nonetheless, this questionnaire is a very useful guide to understanding the amount of attention you may need to focus on the adrenals.

Scoring the questionnaire
Each "yes" answer scores 1 point.

Do you:
1 Often feel tired, despite getting a good night's sleep?
2 Regularly crave salt, salty foods, or sugar?
3 Feel as if everything is a chore, even the things you used to enjoy?
4 Get tired out easily, for example does walking the block feel like a marathon?
5 Have a low sex drive or often abstain from sex because you are too tired?
6 Get bothered or irritated by little things that never used to bother you?
7 Get angry quickly, e.g. road rage, yelling at the kids?

8 Eat or smoke compulsively?

9 Need longer to recover from illness, injury, or trauma than you used to?

10 Sometimes feel it isn't worth making an effort, that everything seems so pointless?

11 Suffer from mild to moderate depression?

12 Suffer from PMS (women only)?

13 Feel worse if you skip meals or don't eat regular meals?

14 Prop yourself up with coffee, cola drinks, and sugary snacks including chocolate?

15 Lose your train of thought easily or find it difficult to make decisions?

16 Experience light-headedness when you stand up quickly?

17 Get absent-minded or find that your short-term memory often fails?

18 Suffer from mood swings?

19 Struggle to get yourself out of bed in the morning?

20 Get an "afternoon low" or energy dip at around 3–4P.M.?

21 Feel more alert after 6P.M. or your evening meal?

22 Take longer to complete tasks than you used to?

23 Appear to have lost muscle tone despite the same levels of activity?

24 Suffer from high (>139 over > 89) or low (<105 over < 65) blood pressure?

25 Have increased body fat around your middle?

26 Suffer from interrupted sleep or insomnia?

27 Spend the whole day rushing from one task to another?

28 Always feel under pressure at work?

29 Exercise for longer than 45 minutes per session six or more times a week, or exercise for longer than 90 minutes per session four or more times a week?

30 Regularly play competitive sports, or take part in competitions?

31 Suffer from chronic pain?

32 Drink more than 3 glasses of alcohol at any one time, more than twice a week?

33 Suffer from phobias or panic attacks?

34 Consider yourself an anxious person?

Total score =   /34 (women)
Total score =   /33 (men)

Interpreting the questionnaire

0–5   Excellent. You feel in control of your life and enjoy a healthy level of stress. However, do make sure you follow the Insulin Factor Diet Plan to support the healthy function of your adrenals.

6–12   Pretty good, but you need to be careful about the way you handle long-term stress. Ensure you balance your protein and carbohydrate intake, and in particular eat some protein at breakfast, as recommended in the Insulin Factor Diet Plan. Any one of the Insulin Resistance Supplement Plans will give your adrenals additional support. Make sure you get regular aerobic exercise, but do not greatly increase your exercise program at this time, as explained in the following chapter.

13–20 Not bad, but this suggests there are some areas of your life where stress may well be affecting your health. Follow the Insulin Factor Diet Plan, exercise moderately, and take steps to address areas of your life that make you feel out of control. Your adrenal hormone balance may be a contributory factor to your Insulin Resistance but any of the Insulin Resistance Supplement Plans will give your adrenals the additional support they need.

21–28 Not good! This suggests that stress is almost certainly affecting your health and contributing to your Insulin Resistance. Follow the Insulin Factor Diet Plan, the appropriate Insulin Resistance Supplement Plan, and also add the Adrenal Support Plan for the first month. You can then redo the Adrenal Stress Questionnaire to determine if you can simply rely on the basic adrenal support included in each of Insulin Resistance Supplement Plans (i.e. when you score under 20). You need to look at your lifestyle and take steps to reduce unnecessary sources of stress in your life. You also need to make sure you are getting appropriate exercise as discussed in chapter 10. Consider taking the Adrenal Stress Profile (ASP) saliva test—see below.

29+   Goodness! Stress is seriously interfering with your health and it is more than likely that it is contributing to your Insulin

Resistance. Follow the Insulin Factor Diet Plan, the appropriate Insulin Resistance Supplement Plan, but also add the Adrenal Support Plan for the first two months. You can then redo the Adrenal Stress Questionnaire to monitor your progress. Only when you score less than 20 can you rely on the basic adrenal support in the Insulin Resistance Supplement Plans. You should also do the Adrenal Stress Profile (ASP) saliva test (see below) to identify if you have high or low cortisol and DHEA. If you proceed with this test at once, then send off the saliva samples before starting any supplement plan and wait for the results. You will then know if you need to follow the Lower Cortisol Supplement Plan or Raise Cortisol Supplement Plan. You need to take a serious look at the sources of stress in your life and begin to make changes as soon as possible. Make sure that you are also taking the appropriate exercise (see chapter 10).

Antianxiety remedy for all

If you are an anxious person, whether or not you scored highly in the questionnaire, I would recommend that you take a fantastic remedy called "200mg of Zen," which contains two naturally occurring amino acids. It isn't a sedative, nor is it addictive or accumulative, but it can really help to stop the mind going around in circles and reduce anxiety. It works well for all kinds of anxiety, including panic attacks, phobias, pre-exam nerves, and so on. While it is included in the Antianxiety Supplement Plan in chapter 14 anybody who suffers from any degree of anxiety would find it helpful.

The higher your questionnaire score, the more you should consider taking the Adrenal Stress Profile (ASP) saliva test. This is because a high score can mean you have high or low cortisol levels and/or low DHEA. What happens in the initial stages of stress is that your adrenals pump out higher levels of the hormones cortisol and DHEA. However, over time, the adrenals become less able to sustain this output, and so levels drop. Everybody has a different threshold at which this occurs. The Adrenal Support Plan is a general plan to support your adrenals, whether high or low cortisol exists, but in severe cases you will get much quicker results if you follow the more specific plans for high or low cortisol.

What is stress?

In general biological terms, stress is defined as the body's reaction to disruptive external forces such as heat, altitude, overload, "threatening" situations, lack of sleep, and so on. This reaction is completely normal, and designed to protect you and your body from a perceived or real threat. Once the stressor has gone, the adrenal hormones should return to normal.

A more biological definition would classify stress as any event that upsets the natural homeostatic balance of the hormones adrenaline, noradrenaline, cortisol, DHEA, and neurotensin. However, under the pressure of modern, busy lifestyles, perhaps the most widely understood definition of stress is an excess of or a vulnerability to the multiple demands of work, time, and psychosocial conflicts that we face on a daily basis. This certainly makes it clear why so many of us feel permanently under pressure.

Factors that contribute to stress

There are a number of factors that contribute to our stress burden and in so doing encourage high levels of cortisol:

Emotions
Lifestyle
Exercise
Diet (refined carbohydrates and stimulants)
Injury and inflammation
Environment

The three stages of stress response

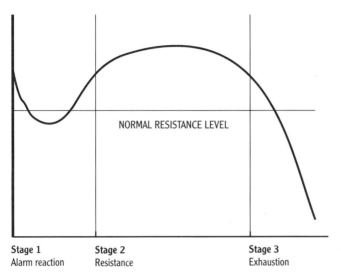

NORMAL RESISTANCE LEVEL

Stage 1
Alarm reaction

Stage 2
Resistance

Stage 3
Exhaustion

There are three stages of stress, based on the research of Dr. Hans Selye, author of *The Stress of Life*, which are helpful to understand the impact of stress on our health.

Stage 1: Alarm reaction

Any physical or mental trauma will trigger an immediate set of reactions. The body releases adrenaline and cortisol and instigates a variety of other psychological mechanisms to combat the stress and help you stay in control. This is called the fight or flight response. The muscles tense, the heart beats faster, breathing rate and perspiration increase, the pupils dilate, and the stomach may clench. This is nature's way of enabling you to either fight or get out of there quick (a response that was obviously of great use to our prehistoric ancestors). But because the body's resources are focused on survival, other systems in the body are put on hold and don't get the resources they need to function optimally. Normally, when the cause of the stress is removed, the body will go back to normal and recover rapidly.

Stage 2: Resistance

If the cause of the stress is not removed, you move into the resistance stage. This is the body's response to what it perceives to be an ongoing threat. It secretes further hormones (e.g. excess cortisol) that increase blood sugar levels to sustain energy and raise blood pressure. A raised cortisol in the short term actually mobilizes the immune system, but in the longer term will ultimately suppress the immune system, lower your levels of resistance, and make you more susceptible to infection and disease. This explains why we initially assume we can resist the effects of stress indefinitely, and believe that we thrive on high levels of stress—because for a short time we can.

During this resistance stage, the hypothalamus (the "master" gland) becomes less sensitive to feedback about the need for stress hormones, resulting in increased cortisol production. Excess cortisol production is associated with a number of metabolic disorders of the hypothalmic-pituitary-adrenal, or HPA, axis (basically the three endocrine glands involved in the stress response), including Insulin Resistance, fat around the middle, higher blood pressure, suppressed immune function, and slow wound healing.

DHEA

We have talked a lot about cortisol, but the role of DHEA is also crucial. DHEA is also a "stress-coping" hormone, and acts as a backup to cortisol by responding to stress and the needs of the immune system. Crucially, however, DHEA reverses immune suppression caused by excess cortisol levels, and therefore improves resistance to viruses, bacteria, yeasts, parasites, allergies, and cancer. It also reverses many other unfavorable effects of excess cortisol and therefore creates improvement in energy, vitality, sleep, PMS, and mental clarity, as well as quicker recovery from any kind of acute stress, excessive mental strain, etc. However, while continued stress raises cortisol levels, it decreases the levels of DHEA. The key to healthy adrenals is therefore to balance both your cortisol and your DHEA levels. The Adrenal Stress Profile (ASP) saliva test will measure both of these.

The DHEA: Insulin connection

DHEA levels are also inversely associated with insulin levels, i.e. when DHEA levels are lower, insulin levels are higher. DHEA can improve blood glucose balance, promote a leaner body, alleviate depression, increase energy, and decrease symptoms of inflammatory conditions such as chronic fatigue, fibromylagia, arthritis, and so on. Many of the problems associated with Insulin Resistance are also associated with low DHEA. This is why it is so important to optimize your DHEA levels.

Stage 3: Exhaustion

The third stage of the General Adaptation Syndrome is exhaustion. In this stage, your body runs out of its reserves of energy and immunity. Your mental, physical, and emotional resources will also be greatly depleted. This is also known as "adrenal exhaustion" or "adrenal burnout." Your blood sugar levels drop as the adrenals become depleted (e.g. low DHEA and low cortisol), leading to decreased stress tolerance, progressive mental and physical exhaustion, illness, and even collapse. Other conditions caused by excessive stress include insomnia, osteoporosis, and a sluggish thyroid.

When your reserves run out you invariably develop a sudden drop in your stress tolerance level, which is why one small event can push you over the edge, as featured famously in the movie *Falling Down* with Michael Douglas, who snaps when he gets stuck in a traffic jam.

The good news is that with the right nutritional program, just as with Insulin Resistance, you can heal your adrenal glands and return to the first stage of adrenal stress. Your body reacts to a stressful situation but afterward your adrenal activity returns to normal.

 Stress is one of the most significant factors lowering your body's resistance to disease and will make you age more quickly, gray hairs and all.

The body's response to stress?

No matter what the source of stress, the body only has one response. Be it a cup of coffee, being late for a meeting, or an emotional upset, the body reacts in the same way, taxing the same system time and again. It is because there are so many things that can cause stress that this response system can become overloaded and exhausted, leading to fatigue, anxiety, depression, insomnia, and, of course, Insulin Resistance.

 No matter what the source of stress, the body only has one response.

Stress, the adrenals, and Insulin Resistance

The adrenal glands are located on top of the kidneys, in the lower back region and secrete the hormones cortisol and DHEA, among others. These adrenal hormones are all too often overlooked when considering Insulin Resistance. Elevated cortisol directly exacerbates Insulin Resistance by preventing insulin from doing its job properly and transporting glucose into cells.

Elevated cortisol directly exacerbates Insulin Resistance.

Conversely, low cortisol and low DHEA reduce your metabolic rate, which is why you often feel tired, crave sugar, and gain weight—and these things alone contribute to Insulin Resistance.

Sometimes changing your diet, exercising regularly, and taking the right supplements won't necessarily resolve Insulin Resistance, and this is invariably because you have an imbalanced level of cortisol and DHEA. For this reason it is important that you examine the impact of stress in your life and take the Adrenal Stress Profile (ASP) saliva test if you scored over 28 in this chapter's questionnaire (and consider taking it if you scored 21–28). As I mentioned earlier, the reason why the saliva test is so important, as opposed to the use of questionnaires alone, is that many of the symptoms associated with high cortisol mimic those of too low a level of cortisol. The Adrenal Support Supplement Plan in chapter 14 is designed to support adrenal function whether the cortisol is high or low, but when you know for sure, you can follow a more targeted supplement plan to address high or low cortisol.

Adrenal Stress Profile test

This test is straightforward to do, involving four simple saliva collections in a single day, and the results are equally simple to interpret. However, if you are in any doubt you should speak to a practitioner familiar with the test (see Resources).

Of all the questionnaires in *The Insulin Resistance Factor*, the Insulin Resistance and Adrenal Stress Questionnaires are the most revealing and relevant to your degree of Insulin Resistance. Once you have completed both, you'll be able to follow the best route to reverse your Insulin Resistance.

Type A personalities, Insulin Resistance, and heart disease risk

Because stress and the body's stress response are so closely tied in with what your mind perceives to be a threat, it is worth considering the kind of person you are and the kind of things that provoke a stress response in you. You may have heard of Type A and Type B personalities, with the former being driven, impatient, and more up-tight than the latter who are more relaxed and carefree. Research has shown that Type A personalities have a distinctly higher risk of suffering from heart disease than Type Bs. This distinction was originally identified by cardiologists who noticed that their patients suffered more anxiety and stress than those with other medical conditions. They went on to discover that people who are generally anxious tend to develop cardiovascular problems.

Type A people are also more prone to Insulin Resistance, so if you can identify yourself as a Type A personality you need to make a conscious effort to change your outlook in life. Obviously, this is not something that will happen overnight, but there are small steps you can take that can reduce unnecessary stress in your daily life and therefore reduce your stress levels. For example, make a list of priorities and get those things done rather than procrastinate with the small stuff. Similarly, if you are the kind of person who worries about being late, allow yourself more time than you actually need to get to your appointment on time. Certain forms of exercise, such as yoga, tai chi, and chi kung, are also very good for helping you manage your anxiety and stress levels (see chapter 10 for more information on suitable exercise). The nutritional support provided by the Insulin Factor Diet Plan and the Supplement Plans will certainly help but in the long term you would be best to address your lifestyle.

Stress and personality type

Particular personality types are more prone to stress than others. These are the so-called "Type A" personalities, people who are hard-driving, competitive, aggressive, impatient, and irritable. Is this due to the effects of high cortisol or the effects of high insulin? Probably both. The more you can identify yourself with Type A, the more you need to offset this with nutritional intervention because it is unlikely that you will be able to change your spots overnight. The following list of traits should help you identify if this is you or not.

Characteristics of a Type A personality pattern

- Hurry sickness—having an ongoing sense of urgency; trying to accomplish too much in too little time.
- Quest for numbers—a preoccupation with ratings, being better than others, earning more money, etc.
- Insecurity of status—having a strong need for "objective" measure of self-worth; pursues achievement to get admiration from others.
- Aggression and hostility—competes with or challenges others continually; struggles to beat others, quick-tempered and angry.
- Rapid and loud speech, replies quickly to questions without deliberation, and finishes other people's sentences.

Summary of key points

▼ Stress is a good thing in the right amounts, but well over half of us suffer from the effects of too much stress.

▼ Stress comes from a variety of sources all of which elicit the same response in the body.

▼ At first stress hormones increase, but with continued stress these hormones decline.

▼ High cortisol is a direct cause of Insulin Resistance, and low DHEA is strongly associated with the condition too.

▼ Stress management is a key factor in Insulin Resistance.

▼ "200mg of Zen" is an excellent and potent natural remedy for anxiety and panic attacks.

▼ The Insulin Factor Diet and Supplement Plans provide general and specific adrenal support.

10 Are You Exercising Enough?

The Insulin Connection

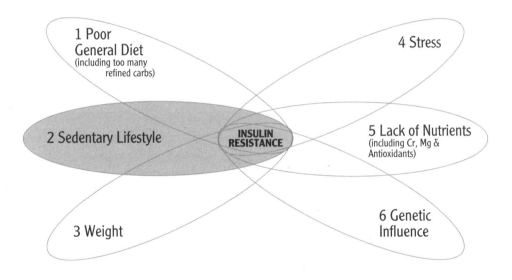

1 Poor General Diet (including too many refined carbs)

4 Stress

2 Sedentary Lifestyle

INSULIN RESISTANCE

5 Lack of Nutrients (including Cr, Mg & Antioxidants)

3 Weight

6 Genetic Influence

"If you lead a sedentary life you run the same risk for cardiovascular disease as those who smoke a pack of cigarettes a day."

Dr. Jim Rippe

The amount of exercise you do on a regular basis is one of the most important influences on the state of your health and your ability to fight against disease. Unfortunately, not all of us exercise enough for some very good reasons, such as work and family commitments, and a minority of us actually get too much exercise, which may be equally harmful as too little.

The quote on the previous page—from Dr. Jim Rippe, former consultant to the US Olympic Team—puts the value of exercise into perspective. The benefits of regular exercise help every system in the body, not least blood glucose and insulin balance. It improves cardiovascular health, bone and muscle mass, lung capacity and circulation, digestive functions, detoxification, immunity, nervous health including stress relief, and helps prevent premature aging. Last but not least, regular exercise helps control weight.

Exercise and Insulin Resistance

You are probably aware that you should exercise, but if you have Insulin Resistance, then you really must exercise regularly—and, most importantly, do the right kind of exercise. Essentially, exercise reduces insulin, helps balance blood glucose, and helps you lose fat and gain muscle. All in all exercise will make you feel and look better. So, what kind of exercise is the right kind? It actually varies from person to person, but generally speaking you need to do moderate cardiovascular or aerobic exercise three to four times a week. This does not mean you have to become a fitness freak, in fact, far from it, because too much exercise will both tax the adrenals and continue to contribute Insulin Resistance. For example, the world's top athletes may be extremely fit but often the intensity and duration of their training is in the long term damaging for their health. A classic example of this is English rowing champion Sir Steve Redgrave, a five-times Olympic gold medalist, who is actually diabetic. Before his diagnosis he would have most certainly been Insulin Resistant, and this would have been brought on by the intensity of his training (causing high levels of oxidative stress and high levels of cortisol) and his need to eat large amounts of food to replenish his lost energy (causing high levels of insulin). Therefore, to excess, exercise increases cortisol levels, sometimes for several hours, and oxidative stress (see chapter 7).

So what is moderate exercise?

Moderate exercise refers to both intensity and duration of what you do. For example, 25 to 40 minutes of cardiovascular exercise at an intensity that causes you to breathe heavily but not gasp for air is moderate. If you are unfit then it won't take a lot to exercise at this level, but as you get more physically fit, you will be able to do more.

Using a heart rate monitor can be very helpful to show you how much you are exerting yourself when you exercise. Generally speaking, you should aim to keep your heart pumping at a rate of 75 percent of your maximum heart rate. To determine this, subtract your age from 220 and multiply by 0.75. For example, a 20-year-old's maximum heart rate is 200, which means an optimum exercise rate of 150. A 50-year-old's maximum heart rate is 170 with an optimum exercise rate of 127.

Exercise, blood glucose levels, and insulin

A newly diabetic client of mine taught me a very important lesson with regard to exercise, blood glucose, and insulin. According to the blood test, he was still producing some insulin, but was progressing to insulin-dependent Type I diabetes. He reported that if he ate lunch and then sat down and did nothing physical his blood glucose would rise quite sharply and he would need to administer insulin to lower it. However, if he went for a walk after lunch he did not need to. What does this tell us? It shows that simply by circulating blood around the body with gentle exercise insulin is more able to dispose blood glucose into muscle and fat tissue than it can when we simply sit still. My client hadn't actually changed his level of fitness, but even this degree of activity helped to reduce his body's need for insulin. This case study shows how useful physical activity of any kind can be in minimizing insulin. However, while a gentle stroll after a meal is a good thing, improving your overall level of physical fitness through regular exercise is markedly more effective at improving insulin's functions. If you remember from chapter 1, muscle tissue is one of the major stores of glucose and the more muscle you have the better able you are to store glucose, minimize insulin and prevent carbohydrates from being converted to fats.

 Going for a walk after a meal helps improve blood glucose and insulin levels; improving your physical fitness is more effective still.

This has been proved in studies between ordinary athletes and people leading a sedentary lifestyle. In one particular study, athletes were able to store 30 percent more glucose and had a 60 percent higher metabolic rate (i.e. they could burn far more calories). What this shows is that someone who is physically fit has a far more effective insulin function than someone who is sedentary.*

What time of day should I exercise?

The best time to exercise is a couple of hours after eating. If you exercise first thing in the morning on an empty stomach, make sure you eat a banana 20 minutes beforehand, and ensure that you also eat afterward to replenish your muscles' energy stores. Avoid exercising late in the evening, particularly if you suffer from insomnia, because this can raise cortisol levels at night, when ideally they should be at their lowest. However, if this is your only opportunity to exercise ensure you exercise gently to moderately to prevent cortisol from being raised for too long afterward. Raised cortisol at night can interfere with sleep and your body's ability to recover on every level. For the same reason, if you can exercise in daylight it's is even better because full spectrum light plays an important role in maintaining the daily rhythm of adrenal hormones.

---

* P. Ebelin, R. Bourey, L. Koranyi, J.A. Tuominen, L.C. Groop, J. Henriksson, M. Mueckler, A. Sovijarvi and V.A. Koivisto, 'Mechanism of enhanced insulin sensitivity in athletes,' *The American Society for Clinical Investigations*, October 1993, 92: 1623–1631.

Exercise and oxidative stress

All exercise causes oxidative stress and this is completely normal because the body requires more oxygen. However, while excess exercise causes excess oxidative stress, moderate exercise actually encourages the body to produce more antioxidant enzymes, so that the net effect of moderate exercise is antioxidative. As mentioned in chapter 7, antioxidants counter the effects of unstable oxygen molecules, or "free radicals," which can damage cells in our bodies. This is another piece of evidence to support moderate exercise over too little or too much.

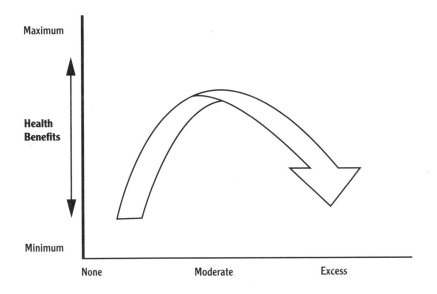

The Insulin Factor 4-Point Exercise Plan

The best type of exercise you can do involves a balance between warming up and down, stretching, resistance work, and cardiovascular exercise. You will require a different balance between these types depending on your degree of Insulin Resistance and the health of your adrenals. You don't have to do all four in one session—though the warming up and down are always recommended—and you can spread them out over the week.

1. Warming up and down

It is important that you warm up before exercise and warm down after exercise, for example, by walking on the spot. You are not aiming to do any stretches at this stage, but rather to prepare the muscles for their workout ahead. Five minutes is fine. Warming the muscles helps prevent injury; warming down helps limit lactic acid buildup and reduce muscle stiffness after you've exercised.

2. Stretching

Stretching exercise does not just include simple flexibility work, but also other forms of exercise such as yoga, tai chi, chi kung, and Pilates. These all involve gentle movement and assuming and maintaining certain positions for a time, often while focusing the mind within the body. While stretching exercises do raise your heart rate it is not what you would call cardiovascular exercise. Stretching helps to focus and relax your mind, so is an excellent form of exercise to counter adrenal stress.

Ensure you learn how to do such exercises safely—I have encountered a number of people who have strained muscles by stretching inappropriately. Stretching properly does not mean bouncing or stretching a muscle to the extent that it hurts. If you are in any doubt, it is always worth joining an exercise class or seeking the help of a personal trainer. Even if you have been exercising independently for years, it may be worth seeking advice to confirm that you are doing it right.

You should aim to stretch for at least 5 minutes before and after any cardiovascular or resistance work. If you are doing yoga, tai chi, Pilates, or other similar forms of stretching exercise, then your session should last between 45 and 90 minutes.

Stretching and the adrenals

In the same way as my client noticed a small but marked improvement when he went for a stroll after eating, stretching exercises do certainly improve your insulin sensitivity but will not have as great an effect as cardiovascular exercise. However, if you scored highly on the Adrenal Stress Questionnaire, you should make this kind of exercise central to your Insulin Factor 4-Point Exercise Plan. This is because stretching exercise will not tax your adrenals or cause as much oxidative stress as cardiovascular exercise exercise would.

3. Cardiovascular exercise

Cardiovascular exercise is also known as aerobic exercise. It is the sort of continuous exercise that makes you huff and puff and perspire. It can also release endorphins and thereby improve mood. It raises your metabolic rate, and improves muscle and heart tone, but does not necessarily increase muscle mass. Any gains in muscle tone that do occur are seen in the early months of training. In fact, if you do too much, you would eventually reduce your muscle mass. Take a look at a marathon runner and you'll see what I mean—they are generally very skinny but actually don't have much muscle.

Examples of cardioivascular exercise

Power walking

Hiking crosscountry

Aerobics machines at the gym

Aerobics classes

Running (preferably not on the hard and polluted roadside)

Cycling to work

Attending dance classes

Swimming

Rowing on the water or on a rowing machine

Walking

Cardiovascular exercise and adrenals

Whenever you do cardiovascular exercise, it elevates adrenal hormones. If you didn't score highly on the Adrenal Stress Questionnaire this is actually fine and you should aim to do cardiovascular exercise for 25–40 minutes three or four times a week. If you did score highly in this questionnaire, then you should limit your cardiovascular exercise to a maximum of 25 minutes twice a week and drop the intensity of your training to 60 percent of your heart rate. Examples of cardiovascular exercise include cycling, running, swimming, crosstraining, ski track, crosscountry skiing, roller blading, aerobics, or playing a sport.

If you scored highly in the Adrenal Stress Questionnaire, you should limit your cardiovascular training to a maximum of 25 minutes twice a week and drop the intensity of your training to 60 percent of your heart rate. This is easy to gauge with a heart rate monitor. For example, a 40-year-old would have a maximum heart rate of 180 (220–40) and so should aim to work out at a heart rate of 108.

4. Resistance

Resistance training, also known as weight or muscle training, forces your muscles to adapt to the challenges placed on them and as a result they become stronger. As we've already said, muscle is one of the main stores of glucose and is much more metabolically active than fat. In this way, resistance training increases your metabolism—you will burn more calories—and improve Insulin Resistance.

If you have Insulin Resistance and didn't score highly in the Adrenal Stress Questionnaire, you should aim to do resistance training two or three times a week for about 30–45 minutes. If you did score highly, then you'll be limiting your cardiovascular exercise and should do more resistance training and stretching (see table opposite for guidance).

Resistance training will increase your heart rate and breathing, but because you rest in between each set of exercises, your heart rate will never be as high as it would with cardiovascular training. The easiest way to do resistance training is at a gym but you can do some exercises at home such as squats, pressups and situps—you may find video or DVD fitness workouts helpful. However, if you are in any doubt about how to do these exercises properly, seek advice from your local gym first. For maximum benefit from resistance training, start by working your largest muscle groups first, such as the leg muscles, chest, and back, and then move on to smaller groups such as the biceps, triceps, and deltoids.

Resistance training and insulin

The more skeletal muscle you have, the greater your insulin sensitivity. Resistance training is the second most important form of exercise for reversing Insulin Resistance.

Resistance training and the adrenals

Regardless of your adrenal status, remember to exercise moderately (i.e. at 75 percent of your maximum heart rate) or, in the case of resistance training, only aim to lift each weight or do each exercise 12 to 15 times. Don't push yourself to the point where you feel you can't possibly do another! Resistance exercises do not have the same relaxing effect on the mind as stretching exercises but it has been shown that the mental activity in the brain does shift from one area to another, thereby reducing stress.

What type of exercise should I emphasize?

Insulin resistant but scored under 21 in the Adrenal Stress Questionnaire

Work at 75 percent of your maximum heart rate.

Type of exercise	Duration and frequency
1 Warmup/warm-down:	5 minutes before and after every exercise session
2 Stretching exercise	45–90 minutes session once a week, and 10–15 minutes 3 times a week
3 Cardiovascular exercise	25–40 minutes, 3–4 times a week
4 Resistance exercise	30–45 minutes, 2–3 times a week

Insulin resistant but scored over 21 in the Adrenal Stress Questionnaire

Work at 60 percent of your maximum heart rate

Type of exercise	Duration and frequency
1 Warmup/warm-down:	5 minutes before and after every exercise session
2 Stretching exercise	45–90 minutes session, 3 times a week, with 2 shorter sessions of 10–15 mins each
3 Cardiocascular exercise	25 minutes, 2 times a week
4 Resistance exercise	30–45 minutes, 3–4 times a week

It may at first be difficult for you to find the time to do this amount of exercise a week, but it really will be worth your while because it will greatly reduce the amount of time needed to reverse your Insulin Resistance. It is better to build up to the weekly optimum number of exercise sessions, rather than follow the plan religiously for one or two weeks then give up on it. If you follow the rest of the plan, it will greatly help your motivation and energy levels and you will actually find it a lot easier to follow than you think.

Caution

If you have been sedentary for some time, it is always worth seeking the advice of a trainer or physiotherapist before you start. They will able to advise you about an exercise plan suitable for your degree of physical fitness.

Summary of key points

▼ Leading a sedentary lifestyle puts you at the same risk of cardiovascular disease as smoking 20 cigarettes a day.

▼ Moderate exercise reduces Insulin Resistance, increases insulin sensitivity, and reduces the risk of heart disease and diabetes.

▼ The more physcially fit you are, the more efficient your insulin becomes at storing glucose.

- If you take a walk after a meal it can reduce your insulin levels.
- Excess exercise increases oxidative stress and speeds aging. Moderation is key.
- Balance your exercise plan to include warming up and down, stretching, and cardiovascular and resistance work.
- If you scored over 21 in the Adrenal Stress Questionnaire, you should limit your cardiovascular work and only exercise at 60 percent of your maximum heart rate.

11 Is It In My Genes?

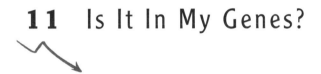

The Insulin Connection

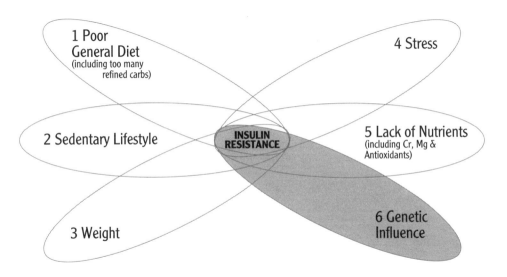

1 Poor General Diet (including too many refined carbs)

4 Stress

2 Sedentary Lifestyle

INSULIN RESISTANCE

5 Lack of Nutrients (including Cr, Mg & Antioxidants)

3 Weight

6 Genetic Influence

The sixth and final cause of Insulin Resistance is your genes, which you may or may not have identified in the Insulin Resistance Questionnaire in chapter 3 as a contributing factor.

Your genetic inheritance can certainly contribute to your risk of Insulin Resistance, but it is usually lifestyle and dietary factors that trigger the genes to contribute more significantly. What this does not mean is that just because there is a history of Insulin Resistance or diabetes in your family you will automatically become insulin resistant or diabetic. Your lifestyle, including how you deal with stress, the amount and type of exercise you do, and the food you eat, all have a much greater influence in the vast majority of cases. Proof of this can be seen in the incidence of diabetes in the world, which has skyrocketed over the last couple of decades. Genes take many hundreds of years to change, so they cannot account for this massive increase. In fact, the actual rate of diabetes is 50,000 times greater than it can be accounted for by genes alone.

 The actual rate of diabetes is 50,000 times greater than it can be accounted for by genes alone.

Who has the most genetic risk?

People who descend from populations that have only more recently, in evolutionary terms, turned to farming and away from a hunter-gatherer existence are most at risk, for example the Arizona Pima Indians, South Asian Indians, Australian Aborigines, New Zealand Maoris, West Indian and Polynesian Islanders, Africans, and Mexicans. This can be explained by what is known as the "thrifty gene," which is life-saving when food supplies are unpredictable, because it helps the body store energy as fat, the most efficient way of storing energy. However, with today's abundance of food this erstwhile protective gene actually works against your health by increasing body fat unnecessarily and at the same time increasing your risk of heart disease, Insulin Resistance, and diabetes. In most cases, health problems did not arise until these groups began eating a Western diet high in refined carbohydrates, omega 6 fats, and trans fats. Insulin Resistance and diabetes were virtually unknown in North American indigenous populations before 1940.*

For example, similarly, South Asians living in the UK have a higher incidence of diabetes than European Caucasians, namely 19 percent as opposed to 4 percent. They also have a significantly greater incidence of

---

* E.J.E. Szathmary, 'Non insulin dependent diabetes mellitus among aboriginal North Americans,' *Ann. Rev. Anth.*, 194, 23: 457–482.

coronary artery disease. The rate is 46 percent higher for men, and 51 percent higher for women. Interestingly, South Asians do not weigh more, but they do tend to gain more fat around their middles. In the USA it is the same story among Asians, Blacks, Hispanics, and Native American Peoples.

Australian Aboriginals

It's a similar scenario for Australian Aboriginals who have developed high rates of obesity, Insulin Resistance, diabetes, and heart disease following the transition from a traditional to an "urbanized" or "Westernized" diet and lifestyle. Of key interest is the fact that there is no diabetes in the Aborigines who have not been "Westernized," indicating that it is a question of how you "nurture" your genes rather than your genes, i.e. nature, alone.

 No matter what your genetic inheritance, you can't change your genes but you can change your diet and lifestyle.

Genes most certainly create differences in disposition to Insulin Resistance between population groups, but the incidence of Insulin Resistance is heavily dependent on diet and lifestyle. Given that we cannot change our genes, anyone in an at-risk group can protect themselves from getting Insulin Resistance and heart disease with the Insulin Factor Diet and Supplement Plans.

Summary of key points

▼ For every individual diagnosed with diabetes there are 4 or 5 who have Insulin Resistance.

▼ The 21st-century epidemic of insulin resistance and diabetes is not purely genetic.

▼ Your genes, particularly the "thrifty" gene, can certainly dispose you to becoming insulin resistant but your diet and lifestyle are what will trigger it.

▼ Caucasians have less genetic disposition to Insulin Resistance than many other ethnicities.

▼ Pima Indians, South Asians, Australian Aborigines, New Zealand Maoris, Native North Americans, African Americans, West Indian and Polynesian Islanders, and Mexicans all have a higher disposition to Insulin Resistance.

Part Four

The Insulin Factor
Plan

12 Your Plan to Reverse Insulin Resistance

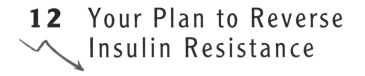

This chapter will help you put together your step-by-step Insulin Factor Plan and start you on the route to reversing Insulin Resistance. It will take your scores from the Questionnaires and show you which of the Insulin Factor Supplement Plans you need to follow. It will also give you an idea of the kind of progress you can expect to make as the weeks go by. Some people will notice immediate improvements, whereas others will notice a more gradual improvement.

As I mentioned at the beginning of the book, there are six main causes of Insulin Resistance and the Insulin Factor Plan will help you address them all.

Reversing Insulin Resistance

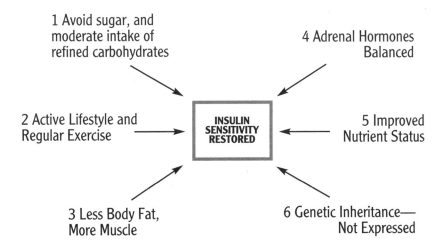

1 Avoid sugar, and moderate intake of refined carbohydrates

4 Adrenal Hormones Balanced

2 Active Lifestyle and Regular Exercise

INSULIN SENSITIVITY RESTORED

5 Improved Nutrient Status

3 Less Body Fat, More Muscle

6 Genetic Inheritance— Not Expressed

Your 5-point action plan

The Insulin Factor Plan consists of five parts:

1 Completing the questionnaires and doing the lab test(s)
2 Diet plan
3 Supplement plans
4 Exercise plan
5 Lifestyle and stress management

Model of how to reverse Insulin Resistance

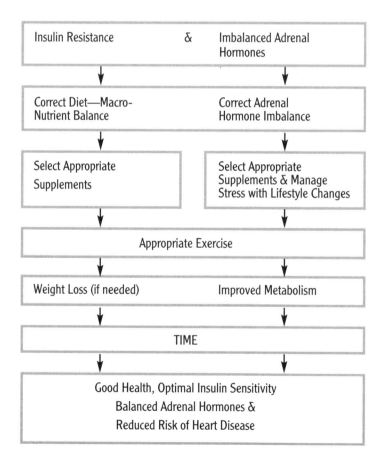

Is there any reason why you shouldn't start immediately?

If you have any medical condition and if you are taking any prescribed drugs it is not recommended you make any changes without first seeking the advice of your healthcare provider.

Even if you do not have a medical condition or take prescription drugs, you may have a physical reason that prevents you from engaging in the complete program. Seek the appropriate medical or other advice on how it may be best for you to proceed.

Step one—Completing the questionnaires and doing the lab test(s)

Start with the Insulin Resistance Questionnaire to establish your degree of Insulin Resistance. Then complete the remaining questionnaires to identify which of the "big six" causes of Insulin Resistance are contributing most to your degree of Insulin Resistance. Obviously, you cannot change your genes, so there are only five areas that you can change.

If you scored more than 21 in either the Insulin Resistance or Adrenal Stress Questionnaires you should consider doing a lab test and now would be a good time to do them (see Resources). However, you can, of course, choose to do these at any time. Insulin and the adrenal hormones are so intimately linked, so it is always worth doing both.

Step two—Diet plan

Start the Insulin Factor Diet Plan in chapter 13, avoiding refined carbohydrates, large meals, stimulants, cigarettes, and excess alcohol.

If your BMI is 30 or more (see chapter 3) make sure that you reduce your carb-protein ratio from 2:1 to 1.5:1. The meal plans provide ratios for each meal, which you should use as a rough guide. For example, if you like the look of a meal but the ratio cited is 2:1, simply reduce the carb portion.

Step three—Supplement plans

Depending on your questionnaire scores you will need to follow certain supplement plans. However, don't worry if you scored highly in all the questionnaires—this doesn't mean you will be rattling with pills from all the supplement plans! If your gut questionnaire score indicated that you need to follow the Gut Supplement Plan you should follow this plan only and none of the others. In a month's time, redo the Gut Questionnaire to see if you still need to follow this plan. If, after two months, there is no improvement, I'd recommend you go and see a practitioner (see Resources).

When you have resolved any problems in your gut, you can then move on to the other supplement plans. However, as I mentioned before, you do not need to follow more than three plans at any one time, even if you scored highly on four or more of the questionnaires.

The table below shows the supplement plans in order of priority. A month after you have started your Insulin Resistance Supplement Plan, and any others, redo the questionnaires to see if you still need to be on the same combination of plans. The majority of people will probably find that they will first need to follow the gut plan, and then a month later start an Insulin Resistance Plan, plus one or two other relevant plans.

Questionnaire or test	Supplement plan	Follow if questionnaire score >	Plan ranking
Gut	Gut Supplement Plan	More than 5	Priority 1
Insulin Resistance (parts 1–4)	Insulin Resistance Supplement Plan 1	22 or less	Priority 2
Insulin Resistance (parts 1–4)	Insulin Resistance Supplement Plan 2	23–40	Priority 2
Insulin Resistance (parts 1–4)	Insulin Resistance Supplement Plan 3	41 or more	Priority 2
Insulin Resistance (Blood Test)	Insulin Resistance Supplement Plan 1, 2 or 3	Depends on test results	Priority 2
Adrenal Stress (Questionnaire)	Adrenal Support Supplement Plan – General	21 or over	Priority 3
Adrenal Stress (Saliva Test)	Adrenal Support Supplement Plan – Lower Cortisol	Depends on test results	Priority 3
Adrenal Stress (Saliva Test)	Adrenal Support Supplement Plan – Raise Cortisol	Depends on test results	Priority 3
Adrenal Stress (Questionnaire)	Antianxiety	21 or more with anxiety	Priority 4
Antioxidant (Questionnaire)	Antioxidant Supplement Plans A, B & C	Plan A: 7 or more Plan B: 17 or more Plan C: 25 or more	Priority 5
Essential Fats (Questionnaire)	Good Fat Supplement Plan A, B, or C	Plan A: 9 or less Plan B: 10–15 Plan C: 16 or more	Priority 6
As needed	Cravings & Appetite Control	As needed	As needed

When do I need to repeat my lab tests?

If you make good progress, redo the Insulin Resistance blood test after three months. If, however, you don't notice any great improvements, then I suggest you redo this test after six weeks to ensure you are on track. The same applies to the Adrenal Stress Profile saliva test.

Should your second test results not show improvements, double check that you are following all relevant parts of the Insulin Factor Plan. Assuming you are, it may simply be a question of time and perseverance. Keep going for another six weeks, redo the tests, and this time, if there is still no improvement, seek the advice of a qualified practitioner (see Resources).

Step four—Exercise plan

Establish which type of exercise described in chapter 10 is most important for your degree of Insulin Resistance and adrenal stress. Start building up to the recommendations below.

The best exercise for you

Insulin resistant but scored under 21 in the Adrenal Stress Questionnaire
Work at 75 percent of your maximum heart rate.

Type of exercise	Duration and frequency
1 Warmup/warm-down	5 minutes before and after every exercise session
2 Stretching exercise	45–90 minutes session once a week, and 10–15 minutes 3 times a week
3 Cardiovascular exercise	25–40 minutes, 3–4 times a week
4 Resistance exercise	30–45 minutes, 2–3 times a week

Insulin Resistant but scored over 21 in the Adrenal Stress Questionnaire

Work at 60 percent of your maximum heart rate.

Type of exercise	Duration and frequency
1 Warmup/warm-down	5 minutes before and after every exercise session
2 Stretching exercise	45–90 minutes session 3 times a week, with 2 shorter sessions of 10–15 minutes each
3 Cardiovascular exercise	25 minutes, 2 times a week
4 Resistance exercise	30–45 minutes, 3–4 times a week

Exercise does not have to be a chore, so look for ways to make it fun and enjoyable. Try and encourage a friend or a member of your family to start exercising with you. The first step toward exercising regularly might seem daunting, but I promise you that once you get into the habit, it will become easier and easier and you will even look forward to it.

Step five—Lifestyle and stress management

If you scored 21 or more in the Adrenal Stress Questionnaire you need to start taking a good look at your lifestyle and see what you can do to reduce any unnecessary sources of stress. As we discussed in chapter 9, making small changes can make all the difference. Stress encourages Insulin Resistance, and if you successfully deal with the one, then the other is more straightforward to solve.

Even if you scored 6 or more you still need to be aware of how stress affects you on a daily basis.

How long will it take before I notice a change in my health?

How much time it takes to reverse Insulin Resistance and make you feel better depends on how overweight you are, your burden of stress, and how easily you can make the dietary and exercise changes.

Generally speaking, you can expect to start feeling better within weeks, sometimes even sooner. For example, some of my clients report a significant change in their food cravings in a couple of days, and find it extremely easy to lose weight as a result. If the Insulin Resistance Supplement Plan doesn't completely get rid of your cravings, then you can always follow the Craving and Appetite Supplement Plan.

That said, it will probably be some months before you can reverse Insulin Resistance, so keep your motivation high by redoing the questionnaires to monitor your progress and looking at that list in the Introduction on pages x–xi showing how good you are going to look and feel when you succeed. If you persevere with the Insulin Factor Plan you most certainly will succeed.

What happens after I have reversed my Insulin Resistance?

Reading this book now, you might not be able to imagine how well you are going to feel when you have reversed Insulin Resistance and your questionnaire scores are low. Believe me—you'll feel fantastic!

To keep feeling like this you should stick with the diet plan long term. If this sounds like a hardship now it won't by the time you have reversed your Insulin Resistance—you'll enjoy your new way of eating too much to be tempted by the thought of your old habits. You'll probably find that you will no longer need to follow the supplement plans but, if you feel that some of the supplements are really helping you stick to the diet plan, don't feel that you have to stop them. As a general rule, I recommend to my "cured" clients that they stick to this diet plan 90 percent of the time and occasionally "indulge" in less insulin-friendly foods. Interestingly, they usually report back that these foods don't hit the spot like they used to!

13 The Insulin Factor Diet Plan

This chapter contains a range of basic recipes and meal plans to get you started on the Insulin Factor Diet Plan. The meal suggestions contain a good ratio of carbs to protein, which is quoted alongside each recipe. Remember, if you have a BMI of 30 or more you need to reduce your portion size of carbohydrates. Initially, feel free to eat more protein because it will help control appetite and cravings, apart from helping minimize insulin. However, in the long term this is not recommended because it creates too much acidity in the body and can also lead to constipation.

All the meals suggested are simple and easy to prepare, which is why I have simply listed the ingredients, and not given a detailed step-by-step preparation guidelines. I'm confident that you will find these meals easy to prepare.

The Insulin-Friendly Food Pyramid

The Insulin-Friendly Food Pyramid below shows you the balance of foods you should eat on a daily basis.

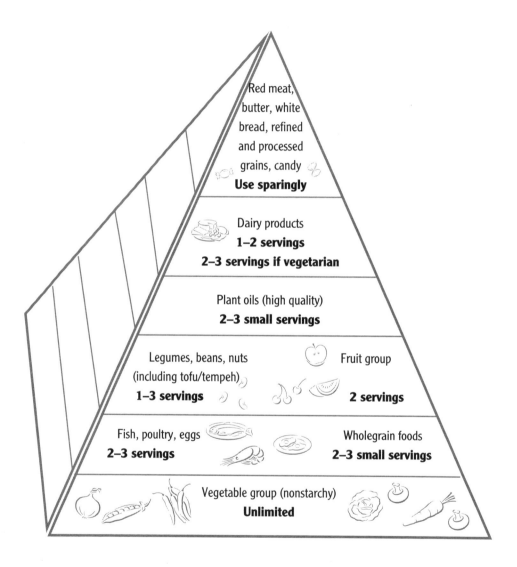

Red meat, butter, white bread, refined and processed grains, candy
Use sparingly

Dairy products
1–2 servings
2–3 servings if vegetarian

Plant oils (high quality)
2–3 small servings

Legumes, beans, nuts (including tofu/tempeh)
1–3 servings

Fruit group
2 servings

Fish, poultry, eggs
2–3 servings

Wholegrain foods
2–3 small servings

Vegetable group (nonstarchy)
Unlimited

A guide to protein portion size

If you have Insulin Resistance you should aim to eat about 1oz (25g) of high BV protein at each meal. The following are examples of suitable protein portion sizes:

Portion size	Amount of protein provided
3 eggs (or 2 whole eggs & 1 white)	¾oz (20g)
Tuna (3oz)	1oz (28g)
Salmon (3oz)	⅘oz (23g)
Sardines (3oz)	⅘oz (23g)
Mackerel (3oz)	⅘oz (23g)
Chicken breast (3oz)	1oz (25g)
Lean meat, fish, poultry (3oz)	¾–1oz (20–25g)
Cottage cheese (½ cup)	¾oz (20g)
Beef steak (3oz)	⅘oz (23g)
Beans 1½ cups + seeds 2–4 tbsp	⅓–¾oz (10–19g) + 1/4–2/3oz (5–10g)

These all contain a high BV protein (except for the beans and seeds)

General healthy eating guidelines

1 Chew your food thoroughly. It is difficult to eat fast when you do this, and it also makes you feel full more quickly.

2 Do not miss a meal. Eat three meals and two snacks a day.

3 Eat high biological value (BV) protein at each meal, and eat the protein at the start of the meal, where possible.

4 Eat some fresh vegetables at lunch and dinner.

5 Eat a maximum of two pieces of fresh fruit daily, in between meals.

6 Eat foods that contain essential fats every day.

7 Add olive oil dressings to your salads.

8 Eat whole, unrefined carbohydrates but always have a moderate to small portion at any one time and do not eat carbohydrates by themselves.

9 Buy organic food where possible. This is more important when buying meat because animals have a tendency to accumulate a lot of toxins in their tissues.

10 Eat a wide variety of different foods over the weeks and months.

11 Drink plenty of water during the day—eight large glasses.

12 At the start of two meals or more a day, eat some raw food.

13 Avoid all sugar and refined carbohydrates.

14 Avoid trans, hydrogenated, and partially hydrogenated fats.

15 Avoid fried and barbecued foods.

16 Reduce and then avoid caffeine altogether for four weeks, after which time it is okay to introduce a low-caffeine tea such as green tea.

17 Avoid artificial sweeteners (they will maintain your taste for sweet foods).

18 Avoid alcohol for the first month. After that, half a glass of wine a day is fine.

19 Reduce and avoid smoking.

20 Reduce and then avoid all other recreational drugs.

Meal suggestions

All the meal suggestions below serve one person and have been designed to take into account your dietary needs to reverse Insulin Resistance. Each suggestion considers:

▼ the Glycemic Index and Glycemic Load
▼ the carbohydrate to protein ratio
▼ the biological value (BV) of the protein in the meal
▼ the fiber content of food

The carbohydrate to protein ratio is listed alongside each recipe, as is the biological value (BV) of the protein, which is listed as "High" or "Sufficient." Where the proteins are listed as "Sufficient" an extra protein option is often provided to enable you to increase with that meal the protein as well as the BV.

Key to recipes

C = Carbohydrates

P = Protein

C:P = Carb to protein ratio

BV = Biological value

Breakfasts

Although it's true that breakfast is the most important meal of the day, we often choose the wrong kinds of food to make it the most insulin-unfriendly meal of the day. Because breakfast generally needs to be quick—most of us are all in a rush getting the kids to school or ourselves to work and so on—we are easily tempted by convenience foods like cereals, which you can pour into a bowl and slosh milk on, or bagels, croissants, and waffles smothered in jam or syrup. Unfortunately these refined carbs all elevate your insulin levels and won't help you reverse Insulin Resistance. What's more, most of them leave you feeling hungry by mid-morning—the initial sugar high you get from them is followed by a drop in blood glucose making you feel hungry—hence late-morning hunger pangs.

Fortunately, there are a number of healthy options that don't take much time to prepare and will see you through comfortably until lunchtime. A protein shake, for example, can take less than a minute to prepare, and you can poach or boil an egg in only a couple of minutes.

Protein powders

Protein powders have become widely available, and I've noticed that most of my clients find it much easier to use them to get the right amount of protein they need, especially at breakfast. When looking for a high-quality protein powder make sure that it does not contain any sugar, artificial sweeteners, colorings, flavorings, or preservatives. The powders are best blended with fruit and milk (of your choice) or yogurt for taste, texture, and consistency. Here are three examples:

Biotics Research	Whey protein isolate	1–2 scoops, 1–2 times per day
Biotics Research	Gam octa pro (soy)	1–2 scoops, 1–2 times per day
Biotics Research	Rice protein concentrate	1–2 scoops, 1–2 times per day

Remember that whey protein has the highest BV of all protein foods (see Resources for how to obtain these protein powders).

Margarines

Only choose margarines that clearly state on their labels that they contain no trans fats or hydrogenated or partially hydrogenated fats. These are usually available from health food stores. Becel and Benecol are two names to look for.

1	2 whole poached eggs plus 1 egg white and a slice of rye or whole-wheat toast, with ⅓ cup mixed berries	C:P Ratio = 1.14 to 1 BV = High Protein = 18g
2	Scrambled eggs (2 whites, 1 yolk) with cilantro, onion, and sweet bell pepper, with either 1 slice of rye toast or ⅓ cup raspberries or strawberries	C:P Ratio = 1.9 to 1 BV = High Protein = 13g
	Protein option: add 1 or 2 more egg whites to scrambled eggs to increase the protein	
3	Porridge made with rolled oats (⅔ cup), milk (skim or soy light) or water, with 1 tbsp natural low-fat yogurt topping and freshly ground sunflower seeds (½ tbsp) Optional extra: add ½ tsp cinnamon to the porridge while cooking	C:P Ratio = 2.9 to 1 BV = Sufficient Protein = 22g
	Protein option: blend 1 heaping tbsp of protein powder into the liquid before cooking the oats in it	C:P Ratio = 2.1 to 1 BV = High Protein = 30g
4	Option A (lower carb) 2oz sliced turkey breast on 1 slice of rye/ whole-wheat toast, with ⅔ cup raspberries and 1 tbsp low-fat natural yogurt	C:P Ratio = 1.09 BV = High Protein = 23.5g
	Option B (higher carb) 2oz turkey breast slices on 2 slices of rye/ whole-wheat toast, with ⅔ cup raspberries and 1 tbsp low-fat natural yogurt	C:P Ratio = 1.47 to 1 BV = High Protein = 26g

5   Option A
2 boiled eggs and 1 egg white with ½ slice of rye   C:P Ratio = 0.93 to 1
or whole-wheat toast, ½ tsp nonhydrogenated   BV = High
margarine and ⅔ cup raspberries   Protein = 16.5g

Option B
2 boiled eggs and 1 egg white with 1 slice of rye   C:P Ratio = 1.35 to 1
or whole-wheat toast, ½ tsp nonhydrogenated   BV = High
margarine, with ⅔ cup raspberries   Protein = 17.5g

6   1 cup sugar-free muesli and 1 cup milk (skim   C:P Ratio = 3.9 to 1
or soy light) and 2 tbsp natural low-fat yogurt   BV = Sufficient
     Protein = 17g

Protein option A: add 1 boiled egg   C:P Ratio = 3 to 1
     BV = High
     Protein = 22.5g

Protein option B: 1 tbsp of soy or rice protein   C:P Ratio = 2.7 to 1
powder mixed in the milk before adding to the muesli   BV = High
     Protein = 25g

7   2 slices broiled organic bacon, ⅓ cup mushrooms,   C:P Ratio = 1.65 to 1
and 2 medium-sized tomatoes on 1 slice of   BV = High
rye toast, with ⅓ cup strawberries   Protein = 17.5g

8   2 slices broiled organic bacon, ⅓ cup mushrooms,   C:P Ratio = 1 to 1
and 2 medium-sized tomatoes on 1 slice of   BV = High
rye toast, with 1 boiled egg and 4 small   Protein = 22g
strawberries

9   ½ cup low-fat cottage cheese, ⅓ cup fresh pineapple,   C:P Ratio = 1.16 to 1
1 tbsp sunflower seeds, and 1 slice of rye   BV = High
or whole-wheat toast   Protein = 20.5g

10	Spinach omelette (1 whole egg and 1 white) with scant ½ cup chopped onions on 1 slice of rye or whole-wheat toast	C:P Ratio = 1.54 to 1 BV = High Protein = 14g
11	2oz quinoa flakes, 1 tbsp sunflower seeds, 1 tbsp almonds and 4 tbsp low-fat natural yogurt. Add boiling water to the quinoa flakes and leave for 5 minutes. It soaks up the water and cooks itself in this time. Add the yogurt (cow or soy), sunflower seeds, and almonds. *Optional extra:* add ½ tsp cinnamon to the quinoa flakes before adding the water	C:P Ratio = 1.54 to 1 BV = Sufficient Protein = 16.5g
12	Option A Protein shake: 1 cup skim milk (or soy light or rice milk), ¾oz protein powder (whey, rice, soy), 1 tbsp low-fat natural yogurt, 1 piece of fruit (pear, small banana) Reduce all portion sizes for smaller shake and less protein Option B Protein shake—as above, but add protein powder to liquid and eat the fruit separately with yogurt	C:P Ratio = 2.14 to 1 BV = High Protein = 31.5g
13	Omelette (2 whole and 2 egg whites) with onion and garlic, with 1 medium-sized tomato, and 1 cup mixed berries	C:P Ratio = 1.95 to 1 BV = High Protein = 20g
14	Cinnamon berry crêpe, made with 2 whole eggs and 1 egg white, 1 heaping tbsp whole-wheat or rice flour or 1 scant tbsp buckwheat flour. Add 1 tsp of cinnamon to the mix before cooking. Use 1 tsp olive oil to grease the skillet. Once cooked, add ½ cup mixed berries and 3 tbsp natural low-fat yogurt and roll up.	C:P Ratio = 1.16 to 1 BV = High Protein = 19g

15 Option A
   Toasted oatbran cinnamon bagel with   C:P Ratio = 1.57 to 1
   nonhydrogenated margarine, with protein   BV = High
   shake (see 12 "Option B" above)   Protein = 31g

   Option B
   Use half the protein powder and fruit   C:P Ratio = 2.6 to 1

16 Shredded wheat and milk (skim or soy light), C:P Ratio = 3 to 1
   with ½ cup natural low-fat yogurt as topping BV = Sufficient
   (limit to twice a week maximum)   Protein = 20g

   Protein option: blend 1 heaping tbsp (15g) protein   C:P Ratio = 1.19 to 1
   powder into the milk before pouring onto cereal   BV = High
   (add a few berries for taste)   Protein = 32.5g

Lunches

Unless the meal already contains a salad of some kind, start each lunch with a small mixed salad, dressed with olive oil and balsamic vinegar (this is included in the calculations).

Salad dressings

Homemade dressings are best—they are easy to make and you control the quality of the ingredients. A simple dressing of best high-quality, cold-pressed olive oil and balsamic vinegar makes a salad more interesting, or you can use walnut oil. If you wish, add garlic, fresh lemon juice, mustard seed, and so on. Store in an airtight container in the fridge. It's best to make small amounts at a time and use them quickly to prevent oxidation of the fats. I use a liquid vitamin E to lengthen the shelf life of oils in my fridge (Bio-E Mulsion by Biotics Research). As soon as I buy them, I add a drop or two to help protect them.

1 Chicken with vegetables
   3½oz chicken breast with   C:P Ratio = 1.05 to 1
   1 cup mangetout peas, ¾ cup chopped broccoli,   BV = High
   4 cherry tomatoes, 1 tsp sunflower seeds, with   Protein = 41g
   3 tbsp cooked brown basmati rice

2 Option A
   Fish and walnut salad   C:P ratio = 1.3 to 1
   2½oz sardines, tuna, or mackerel,   BV = High
   scant ¼ cup walnuts, 2 cups watercress, 4 cherry Protein = 27g
   tomatoes, with a small (1¾oz) baked potato

   Option B
   With a very small (1oz) baked potato   C:P Ratio = 1.13 to 1
                                                    BV = High
                                                    Protein = 27g

3   Chicken salad
     2oz chicken breast with ½ cup   C:P Ratio = 1.39 to 1
     mixed vegetables, 1 tbsp cooked brown   BV = High
     basmati rice or potato   Protein = 31g

4   Baked salmon with vegetables
     4oz baked salmon with 1 cup chopped broccoli   C:P Ratio = 1.13 to 1
     ¼ cup sliced carrots, ½ cup sliced onions,   BV = High
     with small (4in) sweet potato   Protein = 27.5g

5   Cottage cheese salad
     ½ cup low-fat cottage cheese, with salad of   C:P Ratio = 2 to 1
     dark green leaves and 1 brown pita bread   BV = High
                                                       Protein = 21g

6   Tofu stirfry
     ½ cup tofu, small chopped onion, 1 garlic clove, C:P Ratio = 1.85 to 1
     minced, 1 medium-sized tomato, 4 tbsp   BV = Sufficient
     chopped vegetables with the 1 tbsp walnuts,   Protein = 18.5g
     with 4 tbsp cooked brown basmati rice. Dress
     with organic soy sauce.

7   Tempeh/tofu burger
     ⅓ cup tempeh, 1 heaping tbsp cooked lentils,   C:P Ratio = 1.55 to 1
     1 tbsp canned lima beans, 2 tbsp chopped onion, BV = Sufficient
     ⅓ cup grated carrots, ⅓ cup beets blended   Protein = 35g
     together and 1 small brown roll.
     To reduce protein and overall size of meal, choose
     smaller portion

8   Turkey breast with vegetables
     3oz turkey breast and 1 scant cup mixed   C:P Ratio = 1.35 to 1
     steamed vegetables, with 3 tbsp cooked   BV = High
     brown basmati rice   Protein = 31g

9   Omelette

1 whole egg and 1 egg white omelette with   C:P Ratio = 2.15 to 1
minced garlic with 1cup chopped broccoli   BV = High
and 5oz new potatoes   Protein = 17g
Optional: eat fewer potatoes to reduce the carbs

10   Egg and cottage cheese salad   C:P Ratio = 2 to 1

1 sliced hard-boiled egg, ⅓ cup low-fat   BV = High
cottage cheese, 3 cups (about 5oz) mixed lettuce   Protein = 18g
leaves, 3 tbsp cooked brown basmati rice

11   Lamb chops with vegetables and sweet potato   C:P Ratio = 1.25 to 1

2 lamb chops weighing 3oz in total with   BV = High
½ cup peas, ¾ cup carrots, and   Protein = 33g
a very small sweet potato

12   Broiled seafood with mixed vegetables   C:P Ratio = 1.69 to 1

1oz each of scallops, mussels, and shrimp,   BV = High
1 scant cup mixed vegetables, and 2 tbsp cooked   Protein = 25g
brown basmati rice

13   Cottage cheese on crackers   C:P Ratio = 1.32 to 1

¾ cup low-fat cottage cheese, 1⅓ cups   BV = High
steamed chopped broccoli, 1 heaping cup   Protein = 27g
steamed carrot slices, 4 Finn Rye Crisp crackers

14   Broiled trout and crunchy vegetables   C:P Ratio = 1.19 to 1

Broiled 3oz trout with ¼ cup almond flakes,   BV = High
served with 20 green string beans, 1 cup   Protein = 32g
chopped broccoli, and 3½oz new potatoes lightly cooked

15   Quinoa and bean salad   C:P Ratio = 2.73 to 1

Cook 3 tbsp dry quinoa grain in boiling water. Mix   BV = Low
3½oz three bean salad with cooked quinoa and   Protein = 16.5g
add 1 cup crunchy vegetables (sliced carrots,
sliced radish, chopped cauliflower) with light
coating of olive oil dressing

Dinners

Soups

Firstly, it goes without saying that you should avoid packaged and canned soups. Fresh soups are altogether a different thing. Fresh soups are an excellent way to obtain a wide range of nutrients, in a hydrating form. As you may recall, I recommend starting each meal with something raw and fresh, but soup can serve this purpose—as long as it is fresh and not packaged or canned.

Vegetable soups do not contain a high BV protein, and while chicken soup and fish soups are derived from high BV proteins, they do not contain enough to qualify them as a high BV protein. This means that you should not rely on soups to provide you with protein. You should think of them as vegetable intake or both vegetable and carbohydrate intake.

The high water content of soups helps control appetite, because the volume stretches the stomach and triggers receptors that tell your brain you are full. In this way, feel free to use soups to control your appetite, because they are also a very nutritious means of obtaining a wide range of nutrients.

1   Turkey with vegetables and sweet potato
    3oz turkey breast with 1 cup mixed peas, carrots,
    and green string beans, and a heaping ⅓ cup
    mashed sweet potato

    C:P Ratio = 1.5 to 1
    BV = High
    Protein = 30g

2   Salmon with steamed vegetables
    3½oz salmon, baked, with 1 cup mixed
    steamed vegetables (carrots, green and red bell
    peppers, kale, onions, and garlic) and 1 brown roll

    C:P Ratio = 1.13 to 1
    BV = High
    Protein = 31g

3   Sea bass in ginger and black bean sauce
    3½oz sea bass, baked, with 1oz black bean
    sauce, ¾ cup chopped scallions, ¾ cup chopped
    green string beans or mangetout, 1½ tbsp sliced
    ginger root, and 2 tbsp cooked brown basmati rice

    C:P Ratio = 1.31 to 1
    BV = High
    Protein = 26.5g

Option A
Chicken breast with mushrooms and walnut salad   C:P Ratio = 0.66 to 1
3oz chicken breast, ⅔ cup sliced mushrooms,   BV = High
⅓ cup chopped onion, 1 sliced garlic clove (optional),   Protein = 33g
1 tbsp chopped walnuts with 3 cups mixed leaf
salad, and 2½oz new potatoes

Option B
Reduce size of chicken portion and increase potatoes
to increase C:P ratio.

5   Onion and garlic omelette   C:P Ratio = 1.4 to 1
     2 whole eggs and 1 egg white omelette with   BV = High
     ½ cup chopped onions and 1 sliced garlic clove, with   Protein = 22g
     ¾ cup each chopped broccoli and cauliflower, steamed,
     served with 1 brown roll

6   Tofu kebabs with peanut butter sauce   C:P Ratio = 2 to 1
     ½ cup tofu, cubed and skewered along with   BV = Sufficient
     1⅓ cups mushroom pieces and ½ cup green bell   Protein = 18g
     pepper chunks, served with 2 tbsp organic peanut
     butter blended with water for sauce, and
     2 tbsp cooked brown basmati rice

7   Tempeh or tofu steamed stirfry
     ½ cup tempeh or tofu, cubed. Put water in wok and   C:P Ratio = 2.04 to 1
     steam fry with lid on. Add scant ½ cup chopped   BV = Sufficient
     mixed vegetables (carrot, onion, garlic, scallions)   Protein = 20g
     and serve with 2 tbsp quinoa, cooked. Add
     organic soy sauce to taste.

8   Option A
     Halibut with green vegetables and sweet potato   C:P Ratio = 1 to 1
     3oz poached or steamed halibut with scant ½ cup   BV = High
     mangetout, ⅔ cup chopped broccoli, 3 tbsp   Protein = 28g
     peas, and ⅓ cup mashed sweet potato

Option B
To increase the C:P ratio, add more sweet potato

9   Chinese-style beef with vegetables
    2oz beef steak, thinly sliced, stir fried;
    ½ cup kale, ½ cup baby corn and
    1½ tbsp sliced ginger root, steamed.
    Serve with 1 brown roll.

    C:P Ratio = 1.19 to 1
    BV = High
    Protein = 20g

10 Baked plaice in white sauce
    3oz plaice (or haddock), covered with "white"
    sauce (made with whole-wheat flour and low fat
    milk, or soy flour and soy milk) and served with
    ⅓ cup peas, scant ½ cup carrots and a small
    sweet potato

    C:P Ratio = 1.65 to 1
    BV = High
    Protein = 29g

11 Cod and red cabbage
    3oz cod (steamed or baked) with 1 heaping
    cup sliced red cabbage, ⅔ cup chopped onion,
    and 1 cup chopped broccoli, steamed, and
    2½oz new potatoes

    C:P Ratio = 1.33
    BV = High
    Protein = 27g

12 Eastern stir-fry chicken
    3oz sliced chicken breast, stir-fried in Thai
    sugar-free sauce with ¾ cup string beans or
    mangetout, ½ cup chopped onion, 2 tbsp
    chopped garlic, and ¼ cup sliced ginger root,
    served with 3½oz soba buckwheat noodles

    C:P Ratio = 1.66 to 1
    BV = High
    Protein = 26g

13 Veggie burger
    5oz veggie burger (made from tempeh, tofu,
    or soybeans), with 5 cherry tomatoes, on bed of
    2 cups shredded lettuce, served with 1 cup baked
    squash or yam

    C:P Ratio = 2.95 to 1
    BV = Sufficient/Low
    Protein = 18g

Note: The protein BV will vary depending on the ingredients of the veggie burger.
Bind together the ingredients with egg white to increase the protein.

14	Vegetarian stuffed sweet bell pepper 2 medium-sized, sweet red bell peppers, filled with mix of 1 heaping cup ricotta cheese, scant ½ cup chopped onion, 2 cups chopped spinach (or 1 cup chopped kale), 1 sliced garlic clove and 1 tbsp brown basmati rice or quinoa	C:P Ratio = 2 to 1 BV = High Protein = 17g
15	Seafood stirfry (stirfry in small amount of water not oil) 1oz each of three of the following: scallops, shrimps, mussels, crab. With ½ cup mung beans, 3 chopped garlic cloves, 3 tbsp chopped onion, 1¾oz Chinese water chestnuts, and ⅔ cup butter beans	C:P ratio = 1.73 to 1 BV = High Protein = 26g

Insulin-friendly herbs and spices

These herbs and spices have all been proven to have a positive effect on insulin function, so add them to your food wherever possible. For example, add cinnamon to your porridge or baked apples.

Apple pie spice	Cinnamon
Cloves	Bay leaves
Turmeric	

Add your own meal suggestions

Once you have got the hang of the kinds of food you can eat and the ratios of carbohydrate and proteins, feel free to improvise and make up your own recipes.

Snacks

Most snack foods contain sugar, refined carbohydrates, and often trans fats as well. This can make healthy snacking difficult. However, there are a variety of insulin-friendly snacks that you can either prepare in advance or quickly when you want them.

Protein is more difficult to obtain in a snack than anything else, and it is not always possible to choose a high BV protein at such times. The snack suggestions below all contain some form of protein and, in many cases, some essential fats too.

You may recall that calcium can help you lose weight. This is why I've included calcium-rich foods both in the meals above and the snacks below.

Remember to chew your snacks as thoroughly as your main meals.

The snacks contain a variety of foods with different "mouth-feels" to them, which is an important component of a satisfying snack.

Dips

Dips bought from the supermarket or deli are a great favorite with many people—but have you checked out the ingredients in some of them? Avoid those with a lot of additives and go for those that are as "natural" as possible, with the fewest ingredients. Be aware, however, that dips are a deceptively rich source of calories. Taramasalata, full-fat hummus, cream-cheese dips, guacamole, and so on are very high in fat calories and, while they do not upset insulin levels in the way refined carbs do, you should beware of consuming too much if you need to lose weight.

On this basis, small is definitely beautiful. Small quantities of dips, such as low-fat hummus, are fine for mid-morning or mid-afternoon snacks with carrot sticks or rye crackers. They can also be eaten at mealtimes—add them to salads instead of a dressing, or use a small amount to increase the variety and taste of a meal.

15 Snacks

1 Tahini (sesame seed spread), liberally spread on rye crackers or 2 rice cakes, with a sugar-free yogurt

2 Crudites (strips of raw carrot, bell pepper, cucumber, celery) and hummus, with 8 almonds

3 A small pear, 15 almonds or cashews and a sugar-free yogurt

4 A few slim crackers (e.g. rye crackers or thin rice cakes) spread with tahini and topped with some sliced apple

5 A handful of walnut pieces mixed with a small cubed apple, a tablespoon of blueberries and sugar-free yogurt

6 One tablespoon of organic peanut butter blended into a natural yogurt. Add to chilled diced apple or pear for a delicious and refreshing snack

7 Two tablespoons of low-fat cottage cheese with carrot or celery sticks and a tablespoon of sunflower seeds

8 Goat's cheese on a cracker (rye crackers or rice cakes) with 8 sliced red grapes

9 Half a cup of strawberries blended with 2–3oz of silken tofu and served chilled

10 Lettuce-wrapped chicken breast slices × 2, with finely diced crunchy vegetables. (Your food processor has a function for turning whole vegetables into this size in seconds—now is the time to use it!)

11 Half a cup of raspberries with cottage cheese and a teaspoon of sesame seeds

12 Three bean salad, with a tablespoon of sunflower seeds

13 Hard-boiled egg salad with carrot sticks (2 eggs or 1 egg and 2 egg whites)

14 Tuna (1oz) and salad with a plain yogurt and lemon dressing topped with 8 cashews or walnuts

15 Cottage cheese with strawberries and pumpkin seeds

Desserts

As you have probably guessed, the majority of desserts are a diversion off your path to reversing Insulin Resistance. In a strange way they are like the typical modern breakfast—they are usually sugar-fests and will upset your blood glucose and insulin levels. You should aim to give up desserts, other than a yogurt or piece of fruit for example, until you have reversed your Insulin Resistance. If you are finding it difficult to resist your cravings for something sweet after a meal, follow the Craving and Appetite Supplement Plan in chapter 14.

When you have reversed your Insulin Resistance you can indulge occasionally but remember to stick to the 90 percent rule—only have desserts 10 percent of the time!

14 What Supplements Should I Take and When?

This chapter is your guide to which supplements you need to take to help you reverse Insulin Resistance. As you will see there are 11 different supplement plans although, as I have already explained in chapter 12, you will not need to follow more than three at any one time.

The supplement plans are:
1 Gut Supplement Plan
2 Insulin Resistance Supplement Plan 1
3 Insulin Resistance Supplement Plan 2
4 Insulin Resistance Supplement Plan 3
5 Adrenal Support Supplement Plan—General
6 Adrenal Support Supplement Plan—Lower Cortisol
7 Adrenal Support Supplement Plan—Raise Cortisol
8 Antianxiety Supplement Plan
9 Antioxidant Supplement Plans A, B & C
10 Good Fat Supplement Plan A, B & C
11 Cravings & Appetite Control Supplement Plan

Before we look at what each of these involves, it is worth taking a look at supplements in general.

Recommended intakes—RDI

The Reference Daily Intake or Recommended Daily Intake (RDI) serve as a guide to what we should be getting to maintain our health when we are well. They do not take into account biochemical individuality and should certainly not be mistaken as a maximum daily allowance. They are, in fact, very conservative allowances and when you have a metabolic problem, such as Insulin Resistance, you'll actually need well over the RDI for a number of nutrients. Don't worry—there is no risk of overdosing on any nutrient in any of the supplement plans, and in the same way you won't get addicted to any of them.

Why do we need supplements anyway?

Regardless of your state of health, there is a very strong argument for all of us to be taking at least a "good" multivitamin and mineral supplement. This is because of the following:

1 Food is not as nutritious as it once was

▼ There are lower levels of nutrients in soil and food now than there use to be, so even a healthy so-called well-balanced diet won't always provide the vitamins and minerals you need.

▼ The refining and processing of foods depletes nutrients, as does cooking.

▼ Many of us don't eat as well as we know we should.

▼ Certain food choices, lifestyle habits, and environmental factors, such as caffeine, alcohol, smoking, and pollution, reduce the body's ability to absorb nutrients.

▼ As you get older, your body becomes less efficient at using nutrients.

▼ Medical insurance and medical care is very costly; supplements are a form of low-cost health insurance.

2 Modern living and pollution increases our need

▼ Lifestyle factors, such as drinking alcohol, smoking, drug use, hormone therapy, dieting, and even regular exercise, all increase the need for nutrients.

▼ Increased levels of pesticides and herbicides in agriculture:
  ■ increase the toxin burden of the body for which additional nutrients are required for protection
  ■ decrease the uptake of nutrients by plants
  ■ deplete the soil of nutrients and do not renew it

▼ Low levels of nutrients increases the risk of serious diseases such as heart disease, stroke, diabetes, and possibly cancer, making is sensible to get more optimal levels of nutrients.

3 Nutrients in larger doses have benefits

▼ Substantial scientific evidence shows that there can be valuable benefits to health from sensible supplementation with appropriate nutrients, in addition to a well-balanced diet

▼ Specific natural substances can offer an equal or greater effect than their equivalent drug but without the potential side effects

4 Clinical experience

More than a decade of clinical practice convinces me that appropriate supplementation produces health benefits above diet alone.

Quality supplements

Supplements do vary tremendously, so it is important to choose high-quality products. Generally speaking, do not choose the cheapest products—price usually reflects the quality of the product. The recommended supplements in this book are ones that I would recommend to my clients. Most of these are not generally available, so you will need to order them. Details are provided in the Resources.

However, it is important to emphasize that nutritional supplements are not a substitute for a healthy diet. The purpose of recommending them is to achieve swifter results than what diet and exercise can achieve alone.

Insulin Factor Supplement Plans

All supplements should be taken with food unless otherwise stated. Take all supplements toward the end of a meal so that at least some food follows them down.

Please note that B vitamins turn urine a fluorescent yellow color, which is entirely natural and is due to the riboflavin (vitamin B_2).

A special note on calcium supplements

There are many different kinds of calcium supplement available, but the most common are the least well absorbed. The actual calcium from calcium carbonate (i.e. chalk) that is absorbed is very poor when taken on its own, at about 5 percent, and may actually affect how well other nutrients are absorbed too. Choose calcium supplements that contain higher levels of calcium in the form of citrate or ascorbate than they do as carbonate. Other easily absorbed forms of calcium are aspartate and amino acid chelates.

1 Gut Supplement Plan

If you need to follow this program do so before you embark on any of the other supplement plans in this chapter. The following supplements are designed for specific gut problems. To help you identify which supplements you should be taking the typical symptoms are listed with them. Take a maximum of three of the supplements listed, i.e. the ones that are most relevant to you.

Symptoms: Food intolerances, abdominal bloating or pain, long-term use of antibiotics
Function: Gut-lining support, anti-inflammatory, anti-pain, gut-immune support

Allergy Research	Perm A Vite powder	1 tablespoon blended in water or milk 30–40 minutes before a meal, ideally twice daily

Symptoms: Gut pain after eating
Function: Digestive system anti-inflammatory support

Allergy Research	Gastrocort II	2–3 caps before each meal by 15–20 mins

Symptoms: Yeast or candida overgrowth, recent use of antibiotics, taking the contraceptive pill, recent food poisoning, diarrhea, or constipation
Function: Restores friendly bacteria levels to normal

Allergy Research	Lactobacillus GG	1 with breakfast

(As a general rule keep in fridge. However this is not essential—e.g. if traveling away for the weekend simply tear off the blister pack for however many you need.)

Symptoms: Stomach discomfort or pain (not abdominal pain)
Function: Stomach-lining support

Biotics Research	Gastrazyme	2 tabs before each meal

Symptoms: Acidy stomach, heartburn, or hiatal hernia
Function: Natural antacid

Allergy Research	Sano Gastril	Suck 2 lozenges in between meals twice daily & as needed

Symptoms: Excess gas 90 minutes or more after eating, abdominal bloating, smelly stools, food in stools, food intolerances
Function: Helps digest food and supports the pancreas

Biotics Research	Intenzyme Forte	1 with each meal

Symptoms: Yeast or candida overgrowth, thrush, or athlete's foot
Function: Natural antiyeast agent

Biotics Research	Caprin (caprylic acid)	Start on 1 per day and then add one every fourth day until you are taking 2 at each meal

Symptoms: Diarrhea, food poisoning, or parasitic infection
Function: Natural antiparasitic agent

Biotics Research	A.D.P. (oregano oil)	1 at each meal, 1 at bedtime

Symptoms: General excess gas, prone to constipation or diarrhea
Function: Absorbs gas in the gut and promotes more optimal bowel motility

Allergy Research	Gastrocleanse	2–4 capsules on an empty stomach, with a glass of water, once or twice daily—mid-A.M. and mid-P.M.

Symptoms: Constipation or dry, hard stools
Function: Eases constipation and softens stools

Allergy Research	Organic Flax Meal	1 tablespoon, presoaked in water, on empty stomach once or twice daily as needed

2 Insulin Resistance Supplement Plan 1

Biotics Research	GlucoBalance	1 at each meal or food intake If you weigh 110–130 pounds, 4 per day maximum If you weigh 130–154 pounds, 5 per day maximum If you weigh more than 154 pounds, 6 per day maximum
Biotics Research	Lipoic Acid 100mg	1 at breakfast
Allergy Research	Phyllanthus Complex (including milk thistle)	1 at breakfast or lunch

Optional extra calcium—for people whose BMI is over 30 and/or who do not eat dalry products

Allergy Research	Calcium & Magnesium Citrate	1 about 30 minutes before each meal or on empty stomach, 3 times per day

3 Insulin Resistance Supplement Plan 2

Biotics Research	GlucoBalance	1 at each meal or food intake If you weigh 100–130 pounds, 4 per day maximum If you weigh 130–154 pounds, 5 per day maximum If you weigh more than 154 pounds, 6 per day maximum
Biotics Research	Lipoic Acid 100mg	1 at breakfast & dinner
Allergy Research	GlucoFit	1 capsule, 30 minutes before breakfast & dinner

| Allergy Research | Phyllanthus Complex (including milk thistle) | 1 at breakfast & dinner |

Optional extra calcium—for people whose BMI is over 30 and/or who do not eat dairy products

| Allergy Research | Calcium & Magnesium Citrate | 1 about 30 minutes before each meal or on empty stomach, 3 times per day |

4 Insulin Resistance Supplement Plan 3

| Biotics Research | GlucoBalance | 1 at each meal or food intake If you weigh 110–130 pounds, 4 per day maximum If you weigh 130–154 pounds, 5 per day maximum If you weigh more than 154 pounds, 6 per day maximum |

| Biotics Research | Lipoic Acid 100mg | 1 at each meal |

| Allergy Research | GlucoFit | 1 capsule, 30 minutes before breakfast & dinner |

| Allergy Research | Phyllanthus Complex (including milk thistle) | 1 at each meal |

Optional extra calcium—for people whose BMI is over 30 and/or who do not eat dairy products

| Allergy Research | Calcium & Magnesium Citrate | 1 about 30 minutes before each meal or on empty stomach, 3 times per day |

5 Adrenal Support Supplement Plan—General

Allergy Research	Stabilium	4 capsules first thing for 2 weeks, then 2 capsules first thing for 2 weeks
Allergy Research	Biotics Research ADB5 Plus™ 1 at breakfast & lunch	Add hot water to 1 tsp powder in the morning—1–2 cups
Biotics Research	Bio C Plus (Vit C 500mg)	1 mid-morning & mid-afternoon

6 Adrenal Support Supplement Plan—Lower Cortisol

If your total cortisol in the saliva test is less than 60

Biotics Research	Phos Serine Complex	1 caps 30 minutes before bed

If your total cortisol in the saliva test is more than 60

Biotics Research	Phos Serine Complex	1 caps 30 minutes before bed and 1 at lunchtime

If your cortisol is high in the morning or noon (in addition to Phos Serine Complex)

Biotics Research	ADHS	2 at breakfast, 1 at noon

7 Adrenal Support Supplement Plan—Raise Cortisol

If your cortisol is low in the morning or noon or afternoon

Biotics Research	Cytozyme AD	1 at breakfast & lunch

If your total cortisol is too low

Allergy Research	Pantothenic Acid 500mg	1 at breakfast & lunch

N.B. If you are vegetarian replace Cytozyme AD with:

| Allergy Research | Biotics Research ADB5 Plus™ 1 at breakfast & lunch | Add hot water to 1 tsp powder in the morning—1–2 cups per day |

8 Antianxiety Supplement Plan

| Allergy Research | 200mg of Zen | As needed, 1 on empty stomach |

9 Antioxidant Supplement Plan A

| Biotics Research | POA-Phytolens | 1 at breakfast & dinner |

Antioxidant Supplement Plan B

| Biotics Research | POA-Phytolens | 1 at breakfast & dinner |
| Allergy Research | NAC 500mg | 1 mid-morning & mid-afternoon (ideally on an empty stomach) |

Antioxidant Supplement Plan C

Biotics Research	POA-Phytolens	1 at breakfast & dinner
Allergy Research	NAC 500mg	1 mid-morning & mid-afternoon (ideally on an empty stomach)
Allergy Research	CoQ10 100mg	1 at breakfast

Information about these supplements

▼ POA-Phytolens

Phytolens is a water-soluble extract isolated from nonsoy legumes. POA-Phytolens is the most potent antioxidant known. It offers protection from a wide range of free radicals, those from the environment as well as those made in the body and liver.

▼ NAC (500mg)

NAC supports the production of the antioxidant enzyme called "glutathione," which helps with liver detoxification and is the brain's most important antioxidant.

▼ CoQ10 (100mg)

CoQ10 helps utilize oxygen for energy and is also a potent antioxidant. It is often recommended for people with chronic fatigue. It can also help with bleeding gums, gum disease, and heart conditions.

10 Good Fat Supplement Plan A

Allergy Research (Omega 3 Fat)	Super EPA (& DHA)	1 per day with food

Good Fat Supplement Plan B

Allergy Research (Omega 3 Fat)	Super EPA (& DHA)	2 per day with food

Good Fat Supplement Plan C

Allergy Research (Omega 3 Fat)	Super EPA (& DHA)	3 per day with food

Allergy Research (Omega 6 Fat, at a separate meal from the Super EPA)	GLA Borage Oil	1 per day with food

Chapter 6 identified the accessory nutrient L-carnitine that helps fat metabolism. Remember, if you scored more than 10 in the Fats Questionnaire and have a BMI over 25, then you should supplement with L-carnitine for three months, as below.

Biotics	L-Carnitine 300mg	2 capsules on an empty stomach twice daily

N.B. Make sure you are taking a multiple formula, such as Glucobalance, when following this plan. If you are vegetarian and do not wish to take fish oil, replace the Super EPA with Biotics Research Flax Seed Oil capsules in the same doses.

11 Cravings and Appetite Control Supplement Plan

Cravings

Allergy Research	L-Glutamine 500mg	2 caps mid-morning & mid-afternoon with water
Biotics Research	Amino Acid Quick Sorb	10–15 drops under tongue as needed
Allergy Research	Buffered Vit C powder	1 tsp in water on empty stomach twice daily or when you get a craving

Appetite Control

Allergy Research	Glucose Tolerance	1 cap with glass water, 30 mins before 1 or 2 meal(s) a day

(protein, fiber, calcium, L-Carnitine, Garcinia Cambogia, +)

Start with the L-Glutamine and if you find that your cravings aren't reduced, then add the Amino Acid Quick Sorb. If this still doesn't crack your cravings, then add the Buffered Vit C powder. Metaplex is specifically designed to help reduce your appetite before a meal.

Amino Acids for Vegans and Vegetarians

Lysine is often the rate-limiting amino acid in vegetarian foods (see chapter 5) and therefore, by adding lysine to your meals, it can increase the biological value (BV) of meals that don't include a high BV protein food.

Allergy Research	L-Lysine 500mg	1 with meal containing low BV protein foods

If you are vegetarian or vegan, then you should also take a multiamino acid formula with or away from food on a daily basis.

Allergy Research	Free Form Aminos	2 at each meal or 3 on empty stomach twice daily

A Final Word

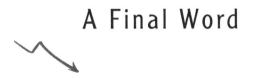

Congratulations!

Once you've got this far with all the changes, you are really on your way to improving your insulin sensitivity. Altering your diet, improving your nutritional status, tackling stress, and incorporating regular exercise is no easy task, so it's quite an achievement. Now, we need to add time to the mix, and watch and wait. The following steps are designed to help you to manage the program once you are into it.

Resources

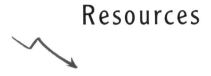

The intention of this section is to enable you to gain access to the tests, the supplements, a practitioner who can help you should you need it, and a number of other related sources of information.

Resource contents

1 Where to find a nutritionist
2 Testing laboratories and the two tests
3 Summary of recommended tests
4 Where to get nutritional supplements
5 BMI table and how to measure BMI
6 Body fat calculations
7 Colleges of nutrition
8 Other information sources
9 Glycemic Index (GI)
10 Index of good sources of essential fatty acids
11 Weights and measures conversion chart

1. Where to find a nutritionist

You are more than welcome to contact myself directly with regard to seeking professional nutritional help and my details are as follows:

Antony Haynes
The Nutrition Clinic
1 Harley Street
London W1G 9QD
Tel: 011 44 626 364 722
Email: antonyjhaynes@aol.com

(clinic only)

Antony Haynes
The Nutrition Clinic
12 Torquay Road, Newton Abbot
Devon TQ12 1AH
Tel: 011 44 626 364 722
Email: antonyjhaynes@aol.com

(all correspondence)

The Nutrition Clinic specializes in the nutritional treatment of Insulin Resistance, founded by the author of this book.

However, in addition, I am pleased to provide a list of nutritionists known to me personally who are trained in and familiar with the subject matter of this book, and whom I would recommend should you need one to one advice. If no one is local to you, please email me on antonyjhaynes@aol.com and I may be able to help you find a nutritionist who is.

Qualified nutritionists

The Institute for Functional Medicine
4411 Pt. Fosdick Drive NW, Suite 305
P.O. Box 1697
Gig Harbor, WA 98335
Tel: (1-800) 228-0622
(253) 858-4724
Fax: (253) 853-6766
client_services@fxmed.com
www.functionalmedicine.org

2. Testing labs

The Insulin Resistance blood test and the Adrenal Stress Profile saliva test can be done via a lab. Call Genova Labs who will direct you to the most local practitioner in your area and then facilitate the test for Insulin Resistence, which is now known as Metabolic Syndrome.

Alternatively, you can also arrange for the test kit to be sent to you and you can have blood drawn locally to where you live (e.g. the doctor's office or local hospital). You then need to ship the blood by courier or express delivery to the lab (the postage would be at your own cost).

Genova Diagnostics
63 Zillicoa Street
Asheville, NC 28801
Tel: (1-800) 522-4762
Local Tel: (828) 253-0621

Adrenal Stress Profile (4 saliva samples) via IWDL—this is one of the few accurate means that exist for determining the degree of stress your body is under, by measuring cortisol and DHEA, over a typical day.

Results take about 10 days to come back.

Call IWDL to arrange the test.

N.B. The IWDL lab is NOT able to provide you with advice about your results, nor make specific recommendations based on your results. However, if you do need to seek the advice of a practitioner, then IWDL can refer you to a qualified nutritionist, or you can refer the list of nutritionists above.

Individual Wellbeing Diagnostic Laboratory (IWDL)
1 Cadogan Gardens
Chelsea
London SW3
Tel: 020 7730 7010 or 020 8336 7750
www.iwdl.net

3. Summary of recommended tests

Degrees of Insulin Resistance

	"Normal"	Stage 1	Stage 2	Stage 3	Stage 4	Diabetes
Fasting Insulin Level	Normal	Normal	Normal	High	High	Lower In time, low
Insulin Levels After a Meal	Normal	High	High	High	High	Low
Triglycerides	Normal	Normal	Higher	High	High	Lower
& HDL	Normal	Normal	Lower	Low	Low	Higher
Body Fat	Normal	Normal	Higher	High	High	Lower
Blood Glucose	Normal	Normal	Normal	Normal	High	Higher

Comparative terms relate to the previous stage on their left.

Insulin Sensitive ⟶ Insulin Resistance ⟶ Diabetes

| Stage 1 | Stage 2 | Stage 3 | Stage 4 | Stage 5 |

The five stages of Insulin Resistance

Stage 1

Insulin levels are raised after eating the "wrong" food (usually high GI carbs), but all other markers are normal.

Action: Follow the Insulin Factor Diet Plan and Insulin Resistance Supplement Plan One.

Stage 2

Insulin levels are high after food, but not when fasting, and you are overweight and you get other symptoms especially after eating refined carbohydrates.

Action: Follow the Insulin Factor Diet Plan and Insulin Resistance Supplement Plan Two.

Stage 3

Insulin levels are now high, fasting and after eating, and triglycerides become elevated and HDL cholesterol goes down.

Action: Follow the Insulin Factor Diet Plan and Insulin Resistance Supplement Plan Three.

Stage 4

Insulin levels are high, as are blood glucose levels, and all of the above.

Action: Follow the Insulin Factor Diet Plan and Insulin Resistance Supplement Plan Three.

Stage 5

Insulin levels become lower, and blood glucose levels are higher still, resulting in diabetes.

Action: Follow the Insulin Factor Diet Plan and follow doctor's drug prescription. Supplements may be appropriate but should be recommended by a qualified nutritionist working with your doctor.

4. Where to get nutritional supplements

UNITED STATES AND CANADA

For people who live in the United States or Canada please call Allergy Research Group LLC, 2300 North Loop Road, Alameda, CA 94502 on (1-800) 545-9960, Worldwide (1-510) 263-2000 and quote "Antony Haynes and *The Insulin Resistance Factor* book" in order to obtain products, or ask for your local Allergy Research Representative. Or, contact Biotics Research Corporation, 6801 Biotics Research Dr., Rosenberg, TX 77471 on (1-800) 231-5777 or Local (281) 344-0909. Ask Biotics Research for your local Biotics Research Representative in order to obtain the products.

UNITED KINGDOM

To make it as easy as possible for you to get the supplements referred to in this book, I have arranged for a single company in the UK to be in a position to provide you with them.

Contact Nutri-Link Ltd, Nutrition House, 24 Milber Trading Estate, Newton Abbot, Devon TQ12 4SG on 08450 760 402; email info@nutri-link.co.uk.

5. BMI table and how to measure BMI

Body Mass Index (BMI) is the measure of body fat based on height and weight that applies to both adult men and women. BMI is intimately related to obesity, because it is a measure of BMI that defines obesity. Obesity has been defined by the National Institutes of Health Consensus Development Conference in 1985 as "an excess of body fat frequently resulting in a significant impairment in health."

BMI is a reliable indicator of total body fat, which is related to the risk of disease and death. The score is valid for both men and women but it does have some limits. The limits are:

▼ It may overestimate body fat in athletes and others who have a muscular build.
▼ It may underestimate body fat in older persons and others who have lost muscle mass.

In and of itself an elevated BMI is a significant risk factor for insulin resistance and heart disease. However, not all obese individuals are insulin resistant or have the metabolic syndrome and not all lean people have insulin that works well (i.e. have insulin sensitivity).

BMI categories:
Underweight = 18.5
Normal weight = 18.5–24.9
Overweight = 25–29.9
Obesity = BMI of 30

We need to work out your BMI because it is important with regard to Insulin Resistance and you will need this figure to complete the questionnaire. Your BMI is combined with other factors relating to your risk for Insulin Resistance in the Insulin Resistance Questionnaire.

Use the BMI table on pages 186–187 to estimate your total body fat.

BMI assessment

For people who are considered obese (BMI greater than or equal to 30) or those who are overweight (BMI of 25 to 29.9) and have two or more risk factors, the guidelines recommend weight loss. Even a small weight loss (just 10 percent of your current weight) will help to lower your risk of developing diseases associated with obesity.

If you need help with assessing your risk, please talk to your doctor who can evaluate your BMI, waist measurement, and others risk factors for heart disease. People who are overweight or obese have a greater chance of developing the cluster of conditions caused at least in part by Insulin Resistance that collectively are referred to as the Metabolic Syndrome: high blood pressure, high blood cholesterol or other lipid disorders, type II diabetes, heart disease, strokes, and certain cancers. Even a small weight loss (just 10 per cent of your current weight) will help to lower your insulin and consequent risk of developing those diseases.

My BMI no.:
Date:

6. Body fat calculations

BMI provides a measure of fatness determined by height and weight, but there is another way of measuring things, one that helps to identify your percentage body fat. Whilst it is BMI that is the official marker for obesity, the Body Fat Calculations may be just as useful. Both can be redone after you have been on the nutritional program for a month in order to monitor progress. Remember that sometimes, weight loss does not always occur first, and this is why other symptom markers as measured by the Insulin Resistance Questionnaire, or the Stress Cortisol Questionnaire would also be useful monitoring tools.

Step 1

Find your body weight (original body weight = OBW), then look on the chart below and then write down the corresponding conversion factor.

For every pound over the nearest figure that you actually weigh add 1.08 to the conversion factor. For example, if your OBW is 175 lbs the conversion factor would be 189.36.

Step 2

Measure your waist girth and then look on the chart below and write down the corresponding number. For example, if your waist girth is 35 inches, the conversion factor would be 145.26. For additional information, if you have a waist that is a quarter of an inch larger than the nearest figure do the following. If the nearest figure is a whole number add 1.04 (total waist size = 37¼ inches add conversion factor 153.56 + 1.04 = 154.60. If the nearest figure is half an inch away, add 1.35. In this example, total waist size = 37¾ add conversion factor 155.63 + 1.35 = 156.98.

Step 3

Subtract the waist conversion factor from the body weight conversion factor (e.g. 189.36 − 145.26 = 44.10).

Step 4

Add the constant of 98.42 for men, or 76.76 for women. (e.g. 44.10 + 98.42 = 142.52). The total represents your lean body weight (LBW).

Step 5

To get your fat weight (FW), follow this equation: OBW − LBW = FW. (e.g. 175 − 142.52 = 32.48).

Step 6

To determine your actual percentage of body fat (BF) follow this equation:

$FW / OBW \times 100 = \%BF$
e.g. $32.48/175 \times 100 = 19\%$

Body Mass Index table

	Normal						Overweight					Obese					
BMI	**19**	**20**	**21**	**22**	**23**	**24**	**25**	**26**	**27**	**28**	**29**	**30**	**31**	**32**	**33**	**34**	**35**

Height (inches)												**Body weight (pounds)**					
58	91	96	100	105	110	115	119	124	129	134	138	143	148	153	158	162	167
59	94	99	104	109	114	119	124	128	133	138	143	148	153	158	163	168	173
60	97	102	107	112	118	123	128	133	138	143	148	153	158	163	168	174	179
61	100	106	111	116	122	127	132	137	143	148	153	158	164	169	174	180	185
62	104	109	115	120	126	131	136	142	147	153	158	164	169	175	180	186	191
63	107	113	118	124	130	135	141	146	152	158	163	169	175	180	186	191	197
64	110	116	122	128	134	140	145	151	157	163	169	174	180	186	192	197	204
65	114	120	126	132	138	144	150	156	162	168	174	180	186	192	198	204	210
66	118	124	130	136	142	148	155	161	167	173	179	186	192	198	204	210	216
67	121	127	134	140	146	153	159	166	172	178	185	191	198	204	211	217	223
68	125	131	138	144	151	158	164	171	177	184	190	197	203	210	216	223	230
69	128	135	142	149	155	162	169	176	182	189	196	203	209	216	223	230	236
70	132	139	146	153	160	167	174	181	188	195	202	209	216	222	229	236	243
71	136	143	150	157	165	172	179	186	193	200	208	215	222	229	236	243	250
72	140	147	154	162	169	177	184	191	199	206	213	221	228	235	242	250	258
73	144	151	159	166	174	182	189	197	204	212	219	227	235	242	250	257	265
74	148	155	163	171	179	186	194	202	210	218	225	233	241	249	256	264	272
75	152	160	168	176	184	192	200	208	216	224	232	240	248	256	264	272	279
76	156	164	172	180	189	197	205	213	221	230	238	246	254	263	271	279	287

Source: Adapted from *Clinical Guidelines on the Identification, Evaluation, and Treatment of Overweight and Obesity in Adults: The Evidence Report.*

36	37	38	39	40	41	42	43	44	45	46	47	48	49	50	51	52	53	54
172	177	181	186	191	196	201	205	210	215	220	224	229	234	239	244	248	253	258
178	183	188	193	198	203	208	212	217	222	227	232	237	242	247	252	257	262	267
184	189	194	199	204	209	215	220	225	230	235	240	245	250	255	261	266	271	276
190	195	201	206	211	217	222	227	232	238	243	248	254	259	264	269	275	280	285
196	202	207	213	218	224	229	235	240	246	251	256	262	267	273	278	284	289	295
203	208	214	220	225	231	237	242	248	254	259	265	270	278	282	287	293	299	304
209	215	221	227	232	238	244	250	256	262	267	273	279	285	291	296	302	308	314
216	222	228	234	240	246	252	258	264	270	276	282	288	294	300	306	312	318	324
223	229	235	241	247	253	260	266	272	278	284	291	297	303	309	315	322	328	334
230	236	242	249	255	261	268	274	280	287	293	299	306	312	319	325	331	338	344
236	243	249	256	262	269	276	282	289	295	302	308	315	322	328	335	341	348	354
243	250	257	263	270	277	284	291	297	304	311	318	324	331	338	345	351	358	365
250	257	264	271	278	285	292	299	306	313	320	327	334	341	348	355	362	369	376
257	265	272	279	286	293	301	308	315	322	329	338	343	351	358	365	372	379	386
265	272	279	287	294	302	309	316	324	331	338	346	353	361	368	375	383	390	397
272	280	288	295	302	310	318	325	333	340	348	355	363	371	378	386	393	401	408
280	287	295	303	311	319	326	334	342	350	358	365	373	381	389	396	404	412	420
287	295	303	311	319	327	335	343	351	359	367	375	383	391	399	407	415	423	431
295	304	312	320	328	336	344	353	361	369	377	385	394	402	410	418	426	435	443

Body fat calculation figures

Body weight	Conversion factor	Waist girth	Conversion factor
100	108.21	25	103.75
105	113.62	25.5	105.83
110	119.03	26	107.90
115	124.44	26.5	109.98
120	129.85	27	112.05
125	135.26	27.5	114.13
130	140.67	28	116.20
135	146.08	28.5	118.28
140	151.49	29	120.35
145	156.90	29.5	122.43
150	162.31	30	124.51
155	167.72	30.5	126.58
160	173.13	31	128.66
165	178.54	31.5	130.73
170	183.95	32	132.81
175	189.36	32.5	134.88
180	194.77	33	136.96
185	200.18	33.5	139.03
190	205.59	34	141.11
195	211.00	34.5	143.18
200	216.41	35	145.26
205	221.82	35.5	147.33
210	227.23	36	149.41
215	232.64	36.5	151.48
220	238.05	37	153.56
225	243.46	37.5	155.63
230	248.87	38	157.71
235	254.28	38.5	159.78
240	259.69	39	161.86
245	265.10	39.5	163.93
250	270.51	40	166.01
255	275.92	40.5	167.08
260	281.33	41	170.16

7. Colleges of nutrition

There are a number of colleges specializing in the training of nutritionists whose graduates practice nutrition. It is always recommended to ask what qualifications a nutritionist has because the term can apply to anyone who has done just a weekend's training, for example. Their course should have lasted for three years, and included relevant clinical skills, not just academic research into nutrient food content. While useful, it does not train someone to be able to provide one to one nutritional advice. Below is a list of colleges offering suitable nutrition courses:

The Institute for Functional Medicine
4411 Pt. Fosdick Drive NW, Suite 305
P.O. Box 1697
Gig Harbor, WA 98335
Tel: (1-800) 228-0622
Local: (253) 858-4724
client_services@fxmed.com
www.functionalmedicine.org

Bastyr University
14500 Juanita Dr. NE
Kenmore, WA 98028-4966
Tel: (425) 823-1300
www.bastyr.edu

8. Other information sources

The Institute for Functional Medicine
4411 Pt. Fosdick Drive NW, Suite 305
P.O. Box 1697
Gig Harbor, WA 98335
Tel: (1-800) 228-0622
Local: (253) 858-4724
client_services@fxmed.com
www.functionalmedicine.org

Bastyr University
14500 Juanita Dr. NE
Kenmore, WA 98028-4966
Tel: (425) 823-1300
www.bastyr.edu

American College of Acupuncture and Oriental Medicine
www.acaom.edu

American College of Homeopathy
www.amcofh.org

American College of Traditional Chinese Medicine
www.actcm.edu

9. Glycemic Index (GI)

The Glycemic Index (GI) is a numerical system of measuring how fast a carbohydrate triggers a rise in circulating blood sugar—the higher the number, the greater the blood sugar response. So a low GI food will cause a small rise, while a high GI food will trigger a dramatic spike. A GI is 70 or more is high, a GI is 56 to 69 inclusive is medium, and a GI of 55 or less is low.

The Glycemic Load (GL) is a relatively new way to assess the impact of carbohydrate consumption that takes the GI into account, but gives a fuller picture than does GI alone. A GI value tells you only how rapidly a particular carbohydrate turns into sugar. It doesn't tell you how much of that carbohydrate is in a serving of a particular food. You need to know both things to understand a food's effect on blood sugar. That is where GL comes in. The carbohydrate in watermelon, for example, has a high GI. But there isn't a lot of it, so watermelon's GL is relatively low. A GL of 20 or more is high, a GL of 11 to 19 inclusive is medium, and a GL of 10 or less is low.

Foods that have a low GL almost always have a low GI. Foods with an intermediate or high GL range from very low to very high GI.

Both GI and GL are listed here. The GL is the GI divided by 100, multiplied by its available carbohydrate content (i.e. carbohydrates minus fiber) in grams. The column showing serving size in grams is required for calculating the GL. Take watermelon as an example of calculating GI. Its GI is pretty high, about 72. According to the calculations by the people at the University of Sydney's Human Nutrition Unit, in a serving of 120 grams it has 6 grams of available carbohydrate per serving, so its GL is pretty low, $72/100 \times 6 = 4.32$, rounded to 4.

The list shows the GI, serving size, and resultant GL.

GI of 70 or more = high	GL of 20 or more = high
GI of 56 to 69 = medium	GL of 11 to 19 = medium
GI of 55 or less = low	GL of 10 or less = low

	Glycemic Index	Serving Size oz (g)	Glycemic Load
Breads			
Baguette, white, plain (France)	95 ± 15	1oz (30g)	15
French baguette with butter, jam	62 ± 7	2½oz (70g)	26
Bagel, white, frozen	72	2½oz (70g)	25
Buckwheat bread, 50% dehusked buckwheat groats & 50% white wheat flour	47	1oz (30g)	10
Melba toast	70	1oz (30g)	16
Gluten-free white bread	71	1oz (30g)	11
Gluten-free fiber-enriched	69	1oz (30g)	9
Bread (45% oat bran, 50% wheat flour)	50	1oz (30g)	9
Rye kernel bread (pumpernickel)	41	1oz (30g)	5
Whole-wheat rye bread (avge)	58 ± 6	1oz (30g)	8
White bread (avge)	70 ± 0	1oz (30g)	10
Whole-wheat bread (avge)	71 ± 2	1oz (30g)	9
Wholegrain wheat bread	46		
Pita bread, white	57	1oz (30g)	10
Flour products			
Banana cake, made with sugar	47 ± 8	3oz (80g)	18
Sponge cake, plain	46 ± 6	2oz (63g)	17
Croissant	67	2oz (57g)	17
Crumpet	69	1¾oz (50g)	13
Doughnut, cake type	76	1½oz (47g)	17
Muffin, apple	44 ± 6	2oz (60g)	13
Muffin, bran	60	2oz (57g)	15
Muffin, oatmeal, made from mix	69	1¾oz (50g)	24
Pancakes, prepared from mix	67 ± 5	3oz (80g)	39
Pastry	59		
Scones, plain, made from mix	92 ± 8	1oz (25)	8
Waffles	76	1¼oz (35g)	10
Breakfast cereals			
All-Bran™ (avge)	42 ± 5		
Bran Flakes™	74	1oz (30g)	13

Cheerios™	74	1oz (30g)	15
Coco Pops™ (avge)	77 ± 3		
Cornflakes™ (avge)	81 ± 3	1oz (30g)	21
Cornflakes, Crunchy Nut™	72 ± 4	1oz (30g)	17
Frosties™ (sugar-coated cornflakes)	55	1oz (30g)	15
Grapenuts™	67	1oz (30g)	13
Alpen Muesli	55 ± 10	1oz (30g)	10
Oat bran, raw	55 ± 5	⅓oz (10g)	2-3
Porridge Oats (avge)	58 ± 4	9oz (250g)	13
Oat porridge (thick dehulled oats)	55	9oz (250g)	15
One Minute Oats	66		
Pop Tarts™, Double Chocolate	70 ± 2	1¾oz (50g)	25
Raisin Bran™	61 ± 5	1oz (30g)	12
Rice Krispies™	82	1oz (30g)	21
Puffed Rice	73		
Shredded Wheat™ (avge)	75 ± 8	1oz (30g)	15
Special K™ (Australia)	54 ± 4	1oz (30g)	11
Special K™ (France)	84 ± 12	1oz (30g)	20
Sultana Bran™	73 ± 13	1oz (30g)	14
Weetabix™	74	1oz (30g)	16

Cereal grains

Amaranth popped	97 ± 19	1oz (30g)	21
Barley, pearled	29		
Barley (avge)	25 ± 1	5¼oz (150g)	11
Buckwheat	63		
Buckwheat (avge)	54 ± 4	5¼oz (150g)	16
Maize flour made into chapatti (India)	59		
Maize meal porridge/gruel (Kenya)	109		
Sweetcorn	62 ± 5	5¼oz (150g)	20
Sweetcorn (avge)	53 ± 4	5¼oz (150g)	17
Couscous (avge)	65 ± 4	5¼oz (150g)	23
Risotto rice (arborio)	69 ± 7	5¼oz (150g)	36
White rice (India)	48	5¼oz (150g)	18
White rice boiled in salted water (India)	72	5¼oz (150g)	27
White rice (Canada)	56	5¼oz (150g)	23
White rice, boiled 13 minutes (Italy)	102	5¼oz (150g)	31

Long grain, white rice	56 ± 7	5¼oz (150g)	24
Long grain, rice boiled 15 mins	58	5¼oz (150g)	23
Long grain, parboiled, 20 mins	75 ± 7	5¼oz (150g)	28
Glutinous white rice (in rice cooker)	98 ± 7	5¼oz (150g)	31
Basmati, white, boiled	58 ± 8	5¼oz (150g)	22
Brown rice (Canada)	66 ± 5	5¼oz (150g)	21
Brown rice, steamed (USA)	50	5¼oz (150g)	16
Instant rice, white, cooked 6 mins	87	5¼oz (150g)	36
Bulgur, boiled 20 minutes (Canada)	53		

Cookies

Digestives	62		
Prince Petit Déjeuner Vanille	45 ± 6	5¼oz (150g)	16
Rich Tea	55 ± 4	1oz (25g)	10

Crackers

Corn thins, puffed corn cakes	87 ± 10	1oz (25g)	18
Puffed crispbread	81 ± 9	1oz (25g)	15
Rice cakes (avge)	78 ± 9	1oz (25g)	17
High-fiber rye crispbread	59	1oz (25g)	9
Rye crispbread	63	1oz (25g)	11
Ryvita	69		
Water crackers (avge)	71 ± 8	1oz (25g)	13

Pasta & noodles

Corn pasta, gluten-free	78 ± 10	6⅓oz (180g)	32
Gluten-free maize pasta, boiled 8 minutes	54	6⅓oz (180g)	22
Fettucine, egg	32 ± 4	6⅓oz (180g)	15
Gnocchi	68 ± 9	6⅓oz (180g)	33
Instant "two-minute" noodles, Maggi®	48 ± 8		
Linguine (avge)	46 ± 3	6⅓oz (180g)	22
Buckwheat noodles	45		
Mung bean noodles (avge)	33 ± 7		
Macaroni (avge)	47 ± 2	6⅓oz (180g)	23
Rice pasta, brown, boiled 16 mins	92 ± 8	6⅓oz (180g)	35
Rice noodles, freshly made, boiled	40 ± 4	6⅓oz (180g)	15
Rice vermicelli	58	6⅓oz (180g)	22

Spaghetti, gluten-free, rice & split pea canned in tomato sauce	68 ± 9	7¾oz (220g)	19
Spaghetti 5 minutes boiled (avge)	38 ± 3	6⅓oz (180g)	18
Spaghetti 15 minutes boiled (avge)	44 ± 3	6⅓oz (180g)	21
Spaghetti white boiled (avge)	42 ± 3	6⅓oz (180g)	20
Whole-wheat spaghetti (avge)	37 ± 5	6⅓oz (180g)	16

Dairy products & alternatives

Ice cream (avge)	61 ± 7	1¾oz (50g)	8
Ice cream, French vanilla, 16% fat	38 ± 3	1¾oz (50g)	3
Ice cream, full-fat (Italy)	11		
Ice cream, full-fat (USA)	40		
Ice cream (avge)	27 ± 4	9oz (250g)	3
Yogurt	36 ± 4	7oz (200g)	3
Low-fat, fruit, sugar, Ski™	33 ± 7	7oz (200g)	10
Whole milk	34		
Skim milk	32		
Soymilk (fat 3%), 120mg Ca	36 ± 4	9oz (250g)	6
Soymilk (fat 1.5%), 120mg Ca	44 ± 3	9oz (250g)	8
Soy yogurt, peach & mango (fat 2%)	50 ± 3	7oz (200g)	13
Tofu-based frozen dessert, chocolate with high-fructose (24%) corn syrup	115 ± 14	1¾oz (50g)	10

Fruit & fruit products

Apple (avge)	38 ± 2	4¼oz (120g)	6
Apple juice, unsweetened (USA)	40	9oz (250g)	12
Apple, dried (Australia)	29 ± 5	2oz (60g)	10
Apricots, dried (Australia)	30 ± 7	2oz (60g)	8
Banana (Canada)	70 ± 5	4¼oz (120g)	16
Banana (Denmark)	46	4¼oz (120g)	12
Banana, underripe	30	4¼oz (120g)	6
Cherries, raw,	22	4¼oz (120g)	3
Cranberry juice drink, Ocean Spray®	56 ± 4	9oz (250g)	16
Dates, dried (Australia)	103 ± 21	2oz (60g)	42
Figs, dried, tenderized	61 ± 6	2oz (60g)	16
Grapefruit, raw	25	4¼oz (120g)	3
Grapes	43–49	4¼oz (120g)	7–9

Kiwi fruit (New Zealand)	47 ± 4	4¼oz (120g)	5
Lychee, canned in syrup	79 ± 8	4¼oz (120g)	16
Mango, ripe (India)	60 ± 16	4¼oz (120g)	9
Marmalade, orange	48 ± 9	1oz (30g)	9
Melon (Cantaloupe)	65		
Oranges (South Africa)	33 ± 6	4¼oz (120g)	3
Orange juice (avge)	52 ± 3	9oz (250g)	12
Paw paw (papaya), ripe (India)	60 ± 16	4¼oz (120g)	17
Peach (avge)	42 ± 14	4¼oz (120g)	5
Peach canned in natural juice (avge)	38 ± 8	4¼oz (120g)	4
Pear (avge)	38 ± 2	4¼oz (120g)	4
Pineapple juice, unsweetened	46	9oz (250g)	15
Pineapple	66		
Plums (avge)	39 ± 15	4¼oz (120g)	5
Prunes, pitted	29 ± 4	2oz (60g)	10
Raisins	64 ± 11	2oz (60g)	28
Strawberries, fresh, raw	40 ± 7	4¼oz (120g)	1
Watermelon, raw	72 ± 13	4¼oz (120g)	4

Weaning foods

Farex™	95 ± 13	3oz (87g)	6

Legumes

Baked beans in tomato sauce	56		
Blackeye beans (avge)	42 ± 9	5¼oz (150g)	13
Chickpeas (avge)	28 ± 6	5¼oz (150g)	8
Kidney beans (avge)	28 ± 4	5¼oz (150g)	7
Kidney beans, dried, soaked 12 h, stored moist 24 hrs, steamed 1 hr (India)	70 ± 11	5¼oz (150g)	17
Lentils (avge)	29 ± 1	5¼oz (150g)	5
Green lentils (avge)	30 ± 4	5¼oz (150g)	5
Red lentils (avge)	26 ± 4	5¼oz (150g)	5
Lima beans	28 ± 7	5¼oz (150g)	5
Mung bean soaked, boiled 20 mins	31	5¼oz (150g)	5
Mung bean, fried	53 ± 8		
Navy beans, boiled (avge)	38 ± 6	5¼oz (150g)	12
Peas, dried, boiled	22	5¼oz (150g)	2

Pinto beans, canned in brine	45	5¼oz (150g)	10
Soybeans, dried, boiled	18 ± 3	5¼oz (150g)	1
Split peas, yellow, boiled 20 mins	32	5¼oz (150g)	6

Nuts

Cashews, salted	22 ± 5	1¾oz (50g)	3
Peanuts (avge)	14 ± 8	1¾oz (50g)	1

Mixed meals and convenience foods

Chicken nuggets, frozen, reheated in microwave oven 5 mins	46 ± 4	3½oz (100g)	7
Fish fingers	38 ± 6	3½oz (100g)	7
Lean Cuisine™	36 ± 6	14oz (400g)	24
Pizza, plain baked dough, served with parmesan cheese & tomato sauce	80	3½oz (100g)	22
Pizza, vegetable supreme, thin & crispy	49 ± 6	3½oz (100g)	12
Stirfried vegetable with chicken & boiled white rice, homemade	73 ± 17	12½oz (360g)	55
Sushi, salmon (from "I Love Sushi")	48 ± 8	3½oz (100g)	17

Snack foods and confectionery

Chocolate, milk, dark with sucrose	34 ± 5	1¾oz (50g)	7
Milk chocolate (avge)	43 ± 3	1¾oz (50g)	12
Chocolate, white, Milky Bar®	44 ± 6	1¾oz (50g)	13
Apricot fruit bar (with whole-wheat pastry)	50 ± 8	1¾oz (50g)	17
Jelly beans (avge)	78 ± 2	1oz (30g)	22
M & M's®	33 ± 3	1oz (30g)	6
Mars Bar®	68 ± 12	2oz (60g)	27
Muesli bar	61		
Nougat, Jijona	32	1oz (30g)	4
Nutella®, chocolate hazelnut spread	33 ± 4	¾oz (20g)	4
Pop Tarts™, double choc	70 ± 2	1¾oz (50g)	24
Power Bar®, chocolate (avge)	56 ± 3	2⅓oz (65g)	24
Snickers Bar®	68	2oz (60g)	23
Skittles®	70 ± 5	1¾oz (50g)	32
Twix®	44 ± 6	2oz (60g)	17

Potato chips, popcorn & corn chips

Corn chips, plain, salted	42 ± 4	1¾oz (50g)	11
Corn chips (avge)	63 ± 10	1¾oz (50g)	17
Popcorn (avge)	72 ± 17	¾oz (20g)	8
Potato chips (avge)	54 ± 3	1¾oz (50g)	11

Soups

Black bean	64	9oz (250g)	17
Lentil, canned	44	9oz (250g)	9
Split pea	60	9oz (250g)	16
Tomato soup	38 ± 9	9oz (250g)	6

Vegetables

Broad beans	79 ± 16	2¾oz (80g)	9
Peas, frozen, boiled (avge)	48 ± 5	2¾oz (80g)	3
Pumpkin	75 ± 9	2¾oz (80g)	3
Corn on the cob, boiled 20 mins	48	2¾oz (80g)	8
Corn (avge)	54 ± 4	2¾oz (80g)	9
Beets	64 ± 16	2¾oz (80g)	5
Carrots, raw	16	2¾oz (80g)	1
Carrots (cooked)	92 ± 20	2¾oz (80g)	5
Parsnips (cooked)	97 ± 19	2¾oz (80g)	12
Potato baked, (avge)	85 ± 12	5¼oz (150g)	26
Boiled white potatoes (avge)	50 ± 9	5¼oz (150g)	14
Canned potatoes (avge)	63 ± 2	5¼oz (150g)	11
French fries, frozen, heated in microwave	75	5¼oz (150g)	22
Instant mash (avge)	85 ± 3	5¼oz (150g)	17
Mashed potato (avge)	74 ± 5	5¼oz (150g)	15
New potatoes (avge)	57 ± 7	5¼oz (150g)	12
Rutabaga	72 ± 8	5¼oz (150g)	7
Sweet potato (avge)	61 ± 7	5¼oz (150g)	17
Tapioca boiled with milk	81	9oz (250g)	14
Yam (avge)	37 ± 8	5¼oz (150g)	13

Indigenous foods

Broken rice, white, cooked in rice cooker (Thailand)	86 ± 10	5¼oz (150g)	37

Glutinous rice, white, cooked in rice cooker (Thailand)	98 ± 7	5¼oz (150g)	31
Udon noodles (avge)	55 ± 7	6⅓oz (180g)	26
Chapatti (Baisen—mixed flours) (avge)	58 ± 9		
Dhokla, leavened, fermented, steamed cake; dehusked chickpea & wheat semolina	35 ± 4		
Idli (parboiled, & raw rice + black dhal, soaked, ground, fermented, steamed) with chutney	60 ± 2	9oz (250g)	31
Laddu (popped amaranth, foxtail millet, roasted legume powder, fenugreek seeds)	29 ± 4		

Pima Indian

Cactus jam (Stenocereus thurberi)	91	1oz (30g)	18

Sugars

Fructose (avge)	19 ± 2	⅓oz (10g)	2
Glucose 2oz (50g) portion (dextrose) (avge)	99 ± 3	⅓oz (10g)	10
Maltose	100		
Honey (avge—11 types)	55 ± 5	1oz (25g)	10
Lactose (avge)	46 ± 2	⅓oz (10g)	5
Sucrose (avge)	68 ± 5	⅓oz (10g)	7
Xylitol	30	1oz (25g)	8 ± 2

Drinks

Coca-Cola® (Australia)	53 ± 7	9oz (250g)	14
Coca-Cola® (USA)	63	9oz (250g)	16
Fanta®	68 ± 6	9oz (250g)	23
Gatorade®	95 ± 10	9oz (250g)	40
Apple juice, unsweetened	40		
Cranberry juice drink, Ocean Spray	56 ± 4	9oz (250g)	16
Orange juice (avge)	50 ± 4	9oz (250g)	13
Pineapple juice, unsweetened	46	9oz (250g)	16
Gatorade®	78 ± 13	9oz (250g)	12
Isostar®	70 ± 15	9oz (250g)	13

10. Index of good sources of essential fatty acids

Omega 3 fats

Where the percentage is given in brackets, this refers to the percentage of the oil contained in the plant that is omega 3, not the percentage of the caloric value.

The best sources of omega 3 fats are from fatty or medium fatty fish, or linseeds. Next come certain nuts and seeds, while legumes, vegetables, and meats contain very low levels.

Fish oils	Plant oils
High	Linseed (flax) (57%)
Salmon (wild)	Linseed meal (14%)
Sardines	Canola (rapeseed) (7%)
Mackerel	Pumpkin (up to 14%)
Tuna	Walnut (5%)
Sea bass	Wheat germ (5%)
Medium	LEGUMES
Trout	Soybeans (7%)
Oysters	Tofu (<5%)
Mussels	
	VEGETABLES
Low	Kale
Cod	Broccoli
Clams	Leafy greens
Flounder	Peas
Halibut	
Scallops	
Shrimps	
Sole	

Omega 6 food sources

Where the percentage is given in brackets, this refers to the percentage of the oil contained in the plant that is omega 6, not the percentage of the caloric value.

The best sources of omega 6 fats are from nut and seed oils, or the nuts and seeds themselves. Next come certain legumes such as soy, whilst vegetables and meats generally contain very low levels.

Plant oils	Nut and seed oils
Safflower (75%)	Sunflower (60%)
Sunflower (60%)	Walnut (51%)
Corn (59%)	Pumpkin (42–57%)
Walnut (51%)	Sesame (45%)
Sesame (45%)	Peanut (29%)
Pumpkin (42–57%)	Brazil (24%)
Soy (50%)	Pecan (20%)
Wheat germ (50%)	Almond (17%)
Canola (30%)	Hazelnut (16%)
Peanut (29%)	Linseed (14%)
Almond (17%)	Cashew (6%)
Linseed (14%)	Coconut (3%)
Olive (8%)	

Legumes and wholegrains	Vegetables
Soybeans	Avocado (10%)
Tofu	
Soymilk	
Legumes (beans, pulses)	
Wheat germ	
Wholegrains (oat, rice, wheat, etc.)	

Omega 9 food sources

Where the percentage is given in brackets, this refers to the percentage of the oil contained in the food that is omega 9, not the percentage of the caloric value.

The most commonly available and best source of omega 9 fat is from olive oil. However, as you will see there are many other oils that contains omega 9 fats, mainly from the nuts and seed family.

Plant oils	Seed and nut oils
Olive (76%)	Almond (78%)
Almond (78%)	Macadamia nut (71%)
Apricot kernel	Cashew (70%)
Avocado (10%)	Pistachio (65%)
Hazelnut (54%)	Pecan (63%)
Rice bran (48%)	Hazelnut (54%)
Pumpkin (34%)	Brazil (48%)
Canola (30%)	Peanut (47%)
Mustard	Sesame (42%)
	Pumpkin (34%)
	Walnut (28%)
	Sunflower (23%)
	Linseed (19%)

Best oils (all fats)	Best margarines (all fats)
Unrefined, extra virgin olive oil	Made from cold-pressed oils
Unrefined safflower/ sunflower oils	Contains NO hydrogenated fats,
Unrefined sesame oil	NO partially hydrogenated fats
Rice bran oil	NO trans fats

11. Weights and measures conversion chart

Imperial	Metric
1oz	28g
2oz	57g
3oz	85g
4oz	113g
5oz	142g
6oz	170g
7oz	198g

Imperial	Metric	Metric	USA
1 teaspoon (0.17oz)	5ml	5 g	1 teaspoon
1 dessertspoon	10ml	10g	2 teaspoons
1 tablespoon (0.5oz)	15ml	14.3g	1 tablespoon
2 tablespoons (1oz)	30ml	28.35g	2 tablespoons
4 fl oz	112.5ml		½ cup
1 teacup (8oz)	1 cup (225g)		225ml
⅘ imperial pint (16oz)	450ml		2 cups (1 pint)
⅘ imperial quart	900ml		1 quart
⅘ imperial gallon	3.6 liters		1 gallon
1 pound	454g		1 pound

Conversion sums

Ounces to grams:

Multiply ounce figure by 28.3 to get number of grams

Grams to ounces:

Multiply gram figure by 0.0353 to get number of ounces

Ounces to milliliters:

Multiply ounce figure by 30 to get number of milliliters

Glossary of Key Words and Terms

Adipose: the scientist's name for fat tissue or body fat.

Adrenaline: one of the major hormones in the body related to stress. It is made in the adrenals and gears the body for fight or flight. It is toxic if it is not "used up."

Advanced Glycation (Glycosylation) End products (AGEs): the resulting product of nonenzymatic modification of macromolecules by glucose. These molecular products may cause pathological changes by changing protein structure, thus altering protein function, cellular transduction pathways, and levels of gene expression. AGE & Hemoglobin-AGE are "late" products of glycation, related to the toxic effects of elevated glucose levels. AGE increase oxidative modification of LDL, which has been suggested to be atherogenic. Antioxidants help protect against the formation of oxidant byproducts from the accumulation of AGE. Modest supplementation of Vitamin E (e.g. 100mg per day) resulted in significantly lower glycosylated hemoglobin and triglyceride levels in Type I diabetic patients. This may link Syndrome X and poor glucose management with the free radical theory of aging first postulated by Denham Harman in 1954.

All cis: in a fatty acid, the configuration where the single hydrogens on both carbons involved in a double bond are found on the same side of the molecule, producing a bend or kink in its shape.

Alpha-linolenic acid (LNA, ALA, 18:3w3): an 18 carbon fatty acid with 3 double bonds, positioned between w carbons 3 and 4, 6 and 7, and 9 and 10. It is the second of two essential fatty acids (EFAs). Our body cannot make it, and requires it for life, and must therefore derive it from food. It is vital for optimal health. It is very sensitive to light, heat, and oxygen. Deficiency is linked to degenerative disease. Modern diets only contain less than one-fifth as much ALA as traditional diets in 1850. ALA inhibits tumor formation. Sources include linseed (flax), and hemp seeds and their oils.

Amino acid: the building block of proteins; there are more than 22 different amino acids present in nature.

Antioxidant: any of a large group of natural or synthetic substances whose presence slows down oxygen- and free radical-induced deterioration of fatty acids and other substances and cells in the body including DNA. Antioxidants are vital to limit oxidative stress that is linked to Insulin Resistance.

Arachidonic acid (AA, 20:4w6): a 20-carbon, 4-time unsaturated fatty acid made from the essential fatty acid linoleic acid by enzymes in our body, and also found in animal foods (meat, eggs, dairy products). It is the parent compound from which pro-inflammatory series 2 prostaglandins are made.

Arteriosclerosis: a thickening of the blood vessel walls and loss of elasticity in small and mid-sized arteries. When arteries lose their elasticity, the flow of blood may become erratic.

Atherosclerosis: the buildup of plaque on the artery walls. The metabolic syndrome increases the rate by which this occurs, which increases blockage risk, which increases heart attack risk, which increases the risk of sudden death.

ATP (adenosine triphosphate): the universal currency of energy used by human cells to provide fuel for biochemical reactions. It is a high-energy phosphate compound that can release large amounts of energy on hydrolysis (addition of water). The vast majority of ATP from ADP (adenosine di-phosphate) is formed in the mitochondria, a process called oxidative phosphorylation, because the oxidation is coupled with the phosphorylation of ADP to form ATP.

Beta carotene: an orange plant pigment constructed of two vitamin A molecules hooked tail to tail. Beta carotene is nontoxic, whereas vitamin A can be toxic. The body stores carotene, and makes vitamin A from it only as it needs vitamin A.

Biochemical toxicology: the biochemical mechanisms that underlie dysfunction or toxicity and that occur primarily at the molecular level.

Carbohydrate sensitivity: describes the small percentage of the population whose internal metabolic reaction to consuming carbohydrates leads to significantly increased fasting insulin levels as well as the insulin response to a glucose tolerance test. In addition, the carbohydrate sensitive individual will have a predisposition to a large and nonadaptable increase in blood triglycerides when they consume diets that are high in carbohydrates, especially sucrose. The lipemia (elevated blood lipids) appears to be carbohydrate related. This genetic disposition is also associated with abnormal glucose tolerance.

Elevated fasting insulin
Elevated 2-hour insulin in GTT
Elevated triglycerides postcarbohydrate intake

Carbon chain: carbon atoms lined to one another in a chain of bonds formed when atoms share electrons.

Cardiovascular disease (CVD): collective term for diseases of the heart and arteries, including arteriosclerosis, atherosclerosis, ischemic heart disease, strokes, heart attacks, high blood pressure, peripheral artery disease, emboli, heart failure, heart enlargement, elevated cholesterol and triglycerides, abnormal blood clotting, and other conditions which now includes hyperhomocysteinemia.

Cell membrane: a double layer of fatty material (phospholipids) and proteins that surrounds each living cell of all organisms.

Cholesterol: a complex fatty substance with many important functions in our body. It can be made in our body or supplied through food of animal origin. Oxidized cholesterol may damage and be deposited in artery linings.

"Cis" in a fatty acid: the natural and good form of an essential unsaturated fat. The arrangement where the single hydrogens on both carbons involved in a double bond are found on the same side of the molecule, producing a bend or kink in its shape.

Citric acid cycle—see Krebs Cycle.

Cold-pressed: Made by first grinding nuts, seeds, fruit, or vegetables into a paste, an oli stone or other tool is used to press the paste which forces the oil to separate out. The oil can not be heated above 80°F during the process.

Complex carbohydrate: sugar-molecules linked together in various ways to make digestible molecules such as starch, and glycogen or indigestible molecules of fiber, which include cellulose, bran, pectin, mucilage, and gum.

Cortisol: adrenal glucocorticoid hormone produced in the adrenal cortex, specifically in the zona fasciculata.

Cytokines: a generic term for all nonantibody proteins released by specific cell types (e.g. macrophages, T lymphocytes) following contact with specific antigens, in order to convey a biological effect within the immune system. Cytokines act as intercellular mediators and as immune-system messenger molecules that can help generate immunoresponsiveness in a variety of tissues. Examples are: IL-1, IL-2, IL-4, IL-6, TNF-a, G-CSF, IFN-a, IFN-y, GM-CSF. Functions of cytokines: intercellular communicators, growth factors for bone marrow stem cells, mediators of antigen processing, plasma cell differentiation, antibody production, modulation of inflammatory response.

Degenerative disease: loss of capacity of cells, tissues, and organs to function normally. Causes include deficiency of essential nutrients, presence of interfering substances, excess of substances, or imbalance in the relative concentrations of substances.

Delta-6-desaturase (D6D): the enzyme that converts w6 linoleic acid (LA) to gammalinolenic acid (GLA) and w3 alpha-loinolenic acid (ALA) to stearidonic acid (SDA).

Deoxyribonucleic acid (DNA): the genetic material that carries the instructions for most living organisms. It is found in two locations in the body: the nucleus of the cell and the mitochondria within cells, the latter of which is inherited entirely from the mother in humans.

Desaturation: the enzymatic process by which 2 hydrogen atoms are removed from neighboring carbon atoms in a fatty acid chain and, at the same time, an additional bond is created between these 2 atoms.

Detoxication: the intracellular biotransformation of endogenous and exogenous toxins into excretable and/ or nontoxic metabolites.

Detoxification: refers to any process used to decrease the negative impact of xenobiotics or toxins on bodily processes. Detoxification therapies may involve many different modalities, including nutritional, botanical, physical, and psychological modalities, and may focus on toxic insult at a number of functional levels, including cellular, organ/tissue specific, or whole body.

DHEA: dehydroepiandrosterone is a steroid hormone, more specifically classified as an adrenal androgen, which has direct biological activity but is best known as a precursor for the active androgenic hormones testosterone and dihydrotestosterone. It plays a role in growth within the body. DHEA is an adrenal cortex hormone, produced in the zona reticularis. Through activity of the enzyme 17-ketosteroid reductase and conversion through androstenediol, DHEA can also be converted into the hormones estrone and estradiol. DHEA is a known inhibitor of the hexose monophosphate shunt, and its secretion is inhibited by insulin. Some studies suggest that insulin has an inverse relationship to DHEA. DHEA has been shown to be antiatherogenic by its inhibition of fibroblasts and its action as a hypolipidemic. The fall in serum levels of DHEA is associated with a higher incidence of atherosclerosis, obesity, and diabetes.

These observations suggest that DHEA may play a role in protection against these disease processes. It has been demonstrated that serum DHEA falls when serum insulin levels rise. Experimentally, induced hyperinsulinemia results in a decline in DHEA sulfate. In vivo studies show that insulin decreases androgen production without affecting adrenal production of glucocorticoids. This is accomplished by inhibiting 17.20 lyase activity (the enzyme involved in the biosynthesis of adrenal androgens), which is a branch point between androgen production and that of glucocorticoids and mineralocorticoids. Thus, insulin reduces serum DHEA by inhibition of production and, to a certain extent, by stimulation of clearance. Clearance is markedly increased for adrenal androgens in obesity, although this appears to play a smaller role.

Dihomogammalinolenic Acid (DGLA, 20:3w6): a fatty acid, the second w6 derivative, made from GLA. DGLA is the parent of the anti-inflammatory hormonelike substances called series 1 prostaglandins, which have many beneficial effects in the body.

Docosahaexanoic acid (DHA, 22:6w3): a 22-carbon fatty acid with 6 double bonds in its chain. It is found in large concentrations in cold-water fish and marine animals, and also in retina, brain, adrenals, and testes. It can be made in health human tissue from the essential alpha-linolenic acid (ALA).

Double bond: a linking of adjacent atoms in the carbon chain by sharing two pairs of electrons between the carbons instead of the usual one shared pair of a single bond.

Dysglycemia: an inability to regulate blood glucose level, associated with irregularities in insulin efficacy and levels. Dysglycemia is associated with the development of NIDDM (noninsulin dependent diabetes aka Type II Diabetes), obesity/excess body fat, hypertension, cardiovascular disease, Syndrome X/Insulin Resistance. Type II diabetes increases risk of heart disease by several-fold, and therefore dysglycemia is associated with the development of cardiovascular disease, which kills more Americans every year than cancer.

Dyslipidemia: resistance to insulin-mediated glucose uptake leads to a compensatory increase in plasma insulin concentration, enhanced hepatic very-low-density lipoprotein (VLDL) and triglyceride (TG) secretion and hypertriglyceridemia.

Eicosanoid: any fatty acid composed of 20 carbons. The most important fatty acid precursor for the eicosanoids is arachidonic acid, a 20-carbon omega-6 fatty acid with 4 double bonds. The highly bioactive families of molecules called prostaglandins, leukotrines, and thromboxanes are all eicosanoids.

Eicosapaentanoic acid (EPA, 20:5w3): a 20-carbon fatty acid with 5 double bonds in its chain. It is found in large quantities in cold-water fish and marine animals. EPA is the parent substance from which the body makes series 3 prostaglandins that decrease inflammation, water retention, and blood pressure by inhibiting the production of pro-inflammatory, water-retaining, artery-constricting series 2 prostaglandins.

Elongation: the enzymatic process by which a fatty acid is lengthened by 2 carbon atoms.

Endocrinology: the study of the endocrine (hormone) system and its role in the physiology in the body.

Enzyme: a protein produced by the body to catalyze particular chemical reactions. An enzyme that catalyzes a reaction is itself not changed.

Essential amino acid: any one of 8 amino acids that the body requires but cannot manufacture and must therefore derive from foods. For children, 10 amino acids are essential. For premature infants, 11 amino acids are essential. Importantly, in various states of unwellness, specific otherwise nonessential amino acids become essential.

Essential fatty acid (EFA): either of 2 fatty acids that the body requires and cannot make from other substances and therefore must derive from the diet. The 2 EFAs are called linoleic acid (LNA) (18:2w6) and Alpha-Linolenic Acid (ALA, 18:3w3).

Essential nutrient: any of more than 45 nutrients that are known to be necessary for body function, structure, and physical health. 20 to 21 minerals, 13 vitamins, 8 to 11 amino acids, and 2 essential fatty acids must form the diet we eat, because the body cannot manufacture them out of other substances or nutrients.

Essential factor: any of about 50 principles known to be necessary for health. In addition to 45 essential nutrients, a source of calorie energy, water, oxygen, and light are included. Sometimes fiber and intestinal bacteria are also included in the list of essential factors.

Expression: the process by which genetic information is transcribed, processed, translated, and ultimately manifested at a phenotypic level. In conventional evolutionary biology, natural selection is viewed as operating on expressed genetic information, rather than on the genetic information itself.

Fat: 3 fatty acid molecules linked to a glycerol molecule in ester links. In layman's terms, it refers to any substances that fit this description and are hard at room temperature because they only contain mostly saturated fatty acids.

Fatty acid: a carbon chain with an organic acid group at one end, and hydrogens attached to the rest of the carbon atoms. The chain length can vary from 4 to 26 or more.

Fiber: any of several indigestible complex carbohydrates that make up the "roughage" or "smoothage" of plant material. They promote bowel regularity, help stabilize blood glucose levels, and help eliminate bile acids, cholesterol, and other waste matter, including hormones, from the body.

Fight/flight response: a sudden release of adrenaline in response to real or perceived stress. Its purpose is to give you the energy to run away from a stressor or fight so that you can survive. When adrenaline is produced and not used up through physical activity, it becomes toxic.

Flax—see linseed.

Free radical: a molecular fragment with a single unpaired electron which, wanting to be paired, steals electrons from other pairs. Free radical reactions occur normally in biological processes. Free radicals are "quenched" by antioxidants, thereby preventing potential cell damage.

Free radical chain reaction: uncontrolled free radical reaction that is damaging to biological processes.

GAS (General Adaptation Syndrome): identified by Dr. Hans Selye, describes the body's mechanism for responding to stress of all different kinds.

Gene: a segment of a DNA molecule (nucleotide sequence) that contains all the information required for synthesis of a product (polypeptide chain or RNA molecule), including both coding and noncoding sequences.

Genotype: the sum total of genetic information contained within an organism.

Glucagon: one of the two main hormones produced by the alpha-cells of the Islets of Langerhans. This hormone promotes glycogen breakdown and protects against hypoglycemia.

Gluconeogenesis: the process of converting other substrates than glycogen to glucose. Sources include lactic and pyruvic acids, and glycerol released by the degradation of triacylglycerol and glucogenic amino acids.

Glucose phosphorylation: the production of ATP from ADP.

Glucose Tolerance Factor (GTF): a combination of chromium, niacin (vitamin B_3), and amino acids. Found in brewer's yeast, GTF improves the body's ability to metabolize glucose, which is vital for minimizing insulin and balancing blood glucose levels.

Glucose transporter proteins: Glut-1, Glut-2, Glut-3, Glut-4—involved in the transportation of glucose into cell.

Glycation: nonenzymatic modification of protein molecules by glucose resulting in abnormal glycosylation.

Glycerol: a molecule that is made up of three carbon atoms, hydrogen, and oxygen. It is the backbone of the fat or oil molecule and of the membranes' fatty components. Two glycerol molecules can be hooked together to make a sugar molecule.

Glycogen: storage form of glucose, usually within the liver and muscle tissue, in the form of glucose molecules hooked together in long chains.

Glycogenesis: formation of new glycogen in liver and muscle tissue.

Glycogenolysis: the process of converting stored glycogen into glucose for use by the brain, red blood cells, and muscle, bone marrow, renal medulla, peripheral nerves. The brain oxidizes glucose completely to CO_2 and H_2O, whereas the other tissues produce lactic or pyruvic acid as a result of glycolysis. This is controlled by insulin and glucagon levels, particularly the ratio of their concentrations.

Glycolysis: the process of energy (ATP) production from glucose. The process even under anaerobic conditions produces two molecules of ATP per mole of glucose, while under aerobic conditions glycolysis produces 38 ATP per mole of glucose.

Hemoglobin AI C: a blood test measuring the percentage of hemoglobin molecules that have been glycosylated (i.e. bound up with a molecule of glucose through a nonenzymatic Amadori chemical reaction). Because red blood cells have a half-life of approximately 120 days, hemoglobin AI C measurement is regarded as an estimate of glycemic control over an approximate three-month period. HgAl C reactions have been determined, however, to be chemically reversible and do not necessarily persist over the lifespan of the red blood cell.

Hemoglobin AGE: a blood test measuring the units of advanced glycation end-products AGEs) per milligram of hemoglobin. Unlike HgAl C, AGE modifications of hemoglobin are chemically irreversible and may better reflect glycemic control. Accumulation of AGE-modified molecules in cells has been associated with oxidative stress reactions and with aging.

High density lipoprotein (HDL): one of the vehicles found in the bloodstream, which carries fats and cholesterol. It returns excess cholesterol from cells to the liver. Our liver changes cholesterol into bile acids, and squeezes them into the intestine to aid with fat digestion on their way out of the body. There are different subtypes of HDL, and LDL, the largest of which is most protective.

Hydrogenation: a commercial process by which liquid oilsare turned into "plastic" or hard fats, by breaking double bonds in fatty acids and forming bonds with hydrogen instead, thereby "saturating" carbon atoms with hydrogen.

Hydrolysis: breakdown of molecules by (enzyme-controlled) addition of a water molecule.

Hyperinsulinism: elevated levels of insulin, usually found in those with Insulin Resistance.

Hypoglycemia: low levels of blood glucose. Can occur after a meal in which case it is referred to as postprandial hypoglycemia or reactive hypoglycemia.

Hypothyroidism: a hormonal condition in which the thyroid gland does not secrete adequate thyroxine to maintain its normal, healthy functions. It is often associated with fatigue and weight gain, although only about 50% of hypothyroid cases are overweight. Can be caused by elevated stress hormone cortisol.

Inflammation: a localized protective response elicited by injury or destruction of tissues, which serves to destroy, dilute, or wall off (sequester) both the injurious agent and the injured tissue.

Impaired Glucose Tolerance (IGT): an inability to regulate blood glucose levels, otherwise referred to as dysglycemia (see above).

Insulin: one of the main hormones produced in the beta-cells of the Islets of Langerhans, which enhances uptake and use of glucose by muscle and adipose tissue. Promotes glycogenesis in liver and muscle, lipogenesis, uptake of glucose by muscle and adipose tissue. Inhibits glycogenolysis (use of glycogen for energy), lipolysis (use of fat for energy). Decreases blood glucose, and increases glycogen and fat stores.

Insulin controls virtually every aspect of growth and metabolism by affecting the transportation of metabolites and intracellular metabolic pathways of most, if not all, of the different cell types in the body. Insulin is a gene expression modulator with influences on a) mitochondrial function, b) cytokine synthesis, c) adrenal and sex hormone metabolism, d) fat mobilization and synthesis. Insulin has major actions in controlling fatty acids and amino acid metabolism too. There is some evidence that insulin also has an action in increasing protein synthesis in some cells. Another important action of insulin is to alter the permeability of cell membranes of a variety of tissues, such as those of the intestine, muscle, and adipose. Insulin stimulates the uptake of carbohydrates and amino acids into these tissues in a selective manner, such that only certain sugars (e.g. glucose or galactose) or amino acids (e.g. alanine) are taken up. The cell membrane carries a specific carrier system for each of these metabolites that requires energy in the form of ATP and that exhibits saturable kinetics: this is called an insulin-sensitive "active transport" mechanism.

Insulin Resistance: a condition in which certain cells do not respond to the normal actions of insulin. Cell receptors do not bind insulin efficiently and therefore the effector action of insulin is partially blunted. In this condition, insulin fails to work effectively in storing blood glucose into muscle or adipose tissue. This leads to an increased blood glucose in the very short term, followed by an increased output of insulin as a compensatory measure in order to maintain normal glucose levels. This results in elevated levels of insulin. Insulin Resistance is the condition which typically precedes, but does not automatically predetermine, NIDDM/Type II Diabetes. This is the central theme of this book.

Insulin sensitivity: this is the normal state in which cells do respond properly to the action of insulin and therefore in a fasting state, at least, normally low levels of insulin are found.

Islets of Langerhans: make up 1–2% of pancreatic tissue. Alpha cells make up 25% of the Islets producing Glucagon, with 50–75% being beta cells that secrete insulin.

Ketone: a breakdown product of fatty acids (FFAs).

Ketosis: a condition characterized by abnormally high levels of ketones in the body. It is a complication of Type I diabetes or prolonged fasting or starvation, or when there are too few carbohydrates in your diet and your insulin effect is too low. In an unrelated subject, a diet which promotes ketosis has been found to be one of the most effective remedial treatments for epilepsy.

Krebs Cycle: the body's main way of releasing the energy stored in chemical bonds, making that energy available for the body's needs. Carbohydrates are its main fuel, but fats and proteins may also be used. It is also called the tricarboxylic acid cycle or citric acid cycle.

Linseed: an ancient plant whose seed is the richest source of alpha-linolenic acid (ALA), which is rare in modern foods. It also contains protein, minerals, and vitamins. It is a rich source of mucilage and fiber, which help the body to eliminate cholesterol and bile acids, and help prevent reabsorption of toxic wastes from the large intestines. Linseed is also the richest source of lignans, which have antiviral, antfungal, antibacterial and anticancer properties. Its oil is used in natural programs for the reversal of cardiovascular disease, cancer, diabetes, premenstrual syndrome, inflammatory conditions, arthritis, and more besides. See Resources for Organic Flax Meal powder, and Organic Flax Seed Oil.

Lipogenesis: the process of storing lipids/fats within adipose tissue.

Lipoprotein(a): an LDL-carrier vehicle of fats and cholesterol, which contains a sticky repair protein known as apo(a), a strong risk factor for cardiovascular disease.

Low density lipoprotein (LD): vehicles that transport fats and cholesterol via the bloodstream to the cells. An excess of these vehicles is said by medical dogma to be associated with cardiovascular disease, hence it is also called the "bad" cholesterol. When measured separately from apo(a), LDL is only a mild risk factor. It is oxidized LDL that poses a much bigger risk factor, and there are at least four subtypes of LDL, the smallest of which are most atherogenic.

Metabolism: all chemical reactions in the body that make physical life possible.

Mitochondria: energy factories of the human cell. They are organelles of 3 um long and 0.5–1 um in diameter. The whole organelle is surrounded by an outer membrane, with an inner membrane forming projections into mitochondrial contents that are called cristae, effectively dividing the mitochondria into a series of compartments. The space between the membranes is termed peripheral space and that between the invaginations the intracristae space.

Mitochondria contain DNA that comes exclusively from the mother, but it cannot code for all of its own proteins. This apparent degree of independence shown by the mitochondria has initiated the proposition that mitochondria were originally bacteria which, long ago, in the course of evolution became assimilated into eukaryotic cells to carry out their oxidative metabolism in a type of symbiosis.

Mitochondria are engaged in effectively trapping energy. The process involves the transformation of energy made available by the oxidation of many molecules normally produced by ingested or stored foods into a form which can be used by the cellular processes. They turn food into ATP, a high-energy phosphate compound. The vast majority of our body's ATP from ADP (adenosine di-phosphate) is formed in the mitochondria, a process called oxidative phosphorylation, because the oxidation is coupled with the phosphorylation of ADP to form ATP.

Mitochondria are oxygen-rich organelles and are thus exposed to free radicals. Interestingly, they lack DNA repair enzymes and are therefore very reliant on antioxidant enzymes such as superoxide dismutase (Mn-SOD, manganese form), lipoic acid, and Coenzyme Q10.

Monounsaturated fatty acid (MUFA): a fatty acid containing one double bond between carbon atoms somewhere in its fatty chain.

Oleic acid (OA): an 18-carbon fatty acid with one double bond between carbons 9 and 10. OA is a monounsaturated fatty acid found in olive, peanut, canola, pecan, macadamia, and other oils.

Omega: symbolized by a w or n, it refers to the methyl end of a fatty acid.

Omega 3 (w or n-3): a family of related polyunsaturated fatty acids essential to human health but lacking from most Western diets. Our intake of these has decreased to one-sixth of their level in 1850. From n-3 fatty acids, our bodies make series 3 prostaglandins, which prevent the negative effects of series 2 prostaglandins by preventing their production.

Omega 6 (w or n-6): a family of related polyunsaturated fatty acids essential to human health and now the dominant type of fat in the Western diet. The parent fat is called linoleic acid (LA), with downstream metabolites including GLA, DGLA, and arachidonic acid. Omega 6 fatty acids are involved in building hormones, being used as cell mediators that increase inflammation (e.g. cytokines), and improve your ability to clot blood and constrict blood vessels.

Oral tolerance: a method of inducing immune tolerance through feeding of low levels of specific protein to produce states of systemic hyporesponsiveness to the fed proteins.

Oxidation: the addition of oxygen, subtraction of hydrogen, or addition of electrons to a substance, often accompanied by a release of energy. This is the reaction from which free radicals, unpaired electrons in the outer shell, are derived. These can then rob other atoms of an electron causing a chain reaction. Oxidation is believed to be the main cause of degenerative disease and aging, in particular premature aging. Antioxidants reduce oxidation in the body.

Phenotype: The observable characteristics of an individual, often regarded as involving the interaction of genotype and environment.

Protein: a group of complex molecules with specific and precise structural and chemical functions. They are made by linking together amino acids (more than 22 different kinds of amino acids are known) in a specific linear sequence and then folding these chains in particular 3-dimensional ways. Enzymes, muscle, and egg white are examples of protein.

Redox potential: the electrochemical potential generated by the presence of a substance that can exist in both oxidized and reduced form. The lower the redox potential of a substance, the greater is its ability to donate electrons. Substances with negative redox potential are therefore, in principle, able to donate electrons to other substances with less negative, zero, or positive redox potential.

SOD: superoxide dismutase is an enzyme of the oxidoreductase class that protects cells against excessive accumulation of superoxide anion radicals by catalyzing the dismutation from two superoxide molecules and two protons to hydrogen peroxide and molecular oxygen. The SOD isoform appearing in the cytosol of the cell requires the metallocofactors copper and zinc. The mitochondrial isoform requires manganese.

Syndrome X: a constellation of interwoven dysfunctions associated with a specialized set of laboratory findings including elevated triglycerides, marginally elevated two-hour postprandial glucose, low HDL, elevated LDL, elevated uric acid, and elevated serum insulin based on oral glucose tolerance testing. Syndrome X is associated with numerous clinical conditions including hyperinsulinemia, adult-onset diabetes, hypertension, hyperlipidemia (elevated triglycerides with low HDL), obesity, breast cancer, strokes, coronary heart diseasem, and polycystic ovary syndrome. Syndrome X manifests as a cluster of symptoms secondary to Insulin Resistance and/or Impaired Glucose Tolerance/dysglycemia. Reference: *Journal of Internal Medicine*, 1994, 236 (suppl. 736): 13–22.

References

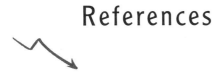

Ahmed A.J., PhD, *Total Health* 23(5):46–48.

Ali L.A., Angyal, G., Weaver, C.M. et al., 'Determination of total trans fatty acids in foods: comparison of capillary-column gas chromatography and single-bounce horizontal attenuated total reflection infrared spectroscopy,' *JAOCS*, 1996; 73:1699–1705.

Ali M. MD, 'Beyond Insulin Resistance and Syndrome X: The Oxidative-Dysoxygenative Insulin Dysfunction (ODID) Model—Part I, II & III,' *Townsend Letter for Doctors & Patients*, August/September, October, November 2002.

Anderson G.H. PhD, Woodend, D. MSc, 'Effect of glycemic carbohydrates on short-term satiety and food intake,' *Nutrition Reviews*, May 2003 (II) 61; 5:S17–S26.

Anderson R.A., 'Recent advances in the clinical and biochemical effects of chromium deficiency.' In A.S. Prasad, ed., *Essential and Toxic Trace Elements in Human Health and Disease: An Update*, New York: Wiley-Liss, 1993:221–234.

Anderson R.A., 'Chromium, glucose tolerance, diabetes, and lipid metabolism,' *J. Advan. Med.*, 1995; 8:37–50.

Anderson R.A., 'Nutritional factors influencing the glucose/insulin system: chromium,' *J. Am. Coll. Nutr.*, 1997; 16:404–410.

Anderson R.A., Bryden N.A., Polansky M.M., 'Strenuous running: Acute effects on chromium, copper, zinc, and selected clinical variables in urine and serum of male runners,' *Biol. Trace Elem. Res.*, 1984; 6:327–336.

Anderson R.A., Bryden N.A., Polansky M.M., 'Dietary chromium intake – freely chosen diets, institutional diets, and individual foods,' *Biol. Trace Elem. Res.*, 1992; 32:117–121.

Anderson R.A., Bryden N.A., Polansky M.M., Reiser S., 'Urinary chromium excretion and insulinogenic properties of carbohydrates,' *Am. J. Clin. Nutr.*, 1990; 1:864–868.

Andres R., 'Aging and diabetes,' *Med. Clin. North Am.,* 1971; 55:835–45.

Arquilla E.R., Packer S., Tarmas W., Miyamoto S., 'The effect of zinc on insulin metabolism,' *Endocrinology,* 1978; 103:1440–1449.

Asayama K., Kooy N.W., Burr I.M., 'Effect of vitamin E deficiency and selenium deficiency on insulin secretory reserve and free radical scavenging systems I islets: decrease of islet manganosuperoxide dismutase,' *J. Lab. Clin. Med.,* 1986; 107:459–464.

Bagchi D., Stohs S.J., Downs B.W., Bagchi M., Preuss H.G., 'Cytotoxicity and oxidative mechanisms of different forms of chromium,' *Toxicology,* 30 Oct. 2002; 180(1):5–22. Comment in *Toxicology,* 2003 Apr. 15;186(1–2), 171–3; author reply 175–7.

Barnard R.J., Roberts C.K., Varon S.M., Berger J.J., 'Diet-induced insulin resistance precedes other aspects of the metabolic syndrome,' *J. Appl. Physiol.,* 1998; 84:1311–1315.

Bergmann J.F., Chassany O., Petit A., Triki R., Caulin C., Segrestaa J.M., 'Correlation between echographic gastric emptying and appetite: influence of psyllium,' *Gut,* 33: 1042–1043.

Bjorntorp P., Rosmond R., 'The metabolic syndrome—a neuroendocrine disorder?,' *Br. J. Nutr.,* Mar 2000; 83 Suppl. 1:S49–57.

Bjorntorp P., Rosmond R., 'Neuroendocrine abnormalities in visceral obesity,' *Int. J. Obes. Relat. Metab. Disord.,* June 2000; 24 Suppl. 2:S80–5.

Blundell J.E., Burley V.J., 'Satiation, satiety, and the action of fiber on food intake,' *Int. J. Obesity,* 11(S1):9–25.

Blundell J.E., Cotton J.R., Delargy H.J., Green S.M., Greenough A., King N.A., Lawton C.L., 'The fat paradox: fat-induced satiety signals versus high fat over consumption.' *Int. J. Obesity,* 19:832–835.

Bonora E., Kiechi S., Willeit J., et al., 'Prevalence of insulin resistance in metabolic disorders: The Bruneck Study,' *Diabetes,* 1998; 47:1643–9.

Brand-Miller J.C. PhD, 'Glycemic load and chronic disease,' *Nutrition Reviews,* May 2003, (II) 61; 5:S49–S55.

Brand-Miller J.C., Holt S.H., Pawlak D.B., McMillan J., 'Glycemic index and obesity,' *J. Am. J. Clin. Nutr.,* July 2002; 76(1):281S–5S.

Bray G.A., Bouchard C., James W.P., 'Handbook of obesity,' New York, NY, Marcel Dekker, Inc, 1998.

Broadhurst C.L. PhD, 'Nutrition & noninsulin dependent diabetes mellitus from an anthropological perspective,' *Alternative Medicine Review,* 1997; 2(5):378–399.

Broadhurst C.L., Cunnance S.C., Crawford M.C., 'Rift Valley lake fish and shellfish provided brain-specific nutrition for early homo,' *Br. J. Nutr.*, in press 1998.

Broughton D.L., Taylor R., 'Deterioration of glucose tolerance with age: the role of Insulin Resistance,' *Age & Aging*, 1991; 20:221–225.

Brownstein D., *Bio-Review*, Newsletter for the healthcare professional, Vol. 1, No.1, 2002.

Burkitt, D. CMG, FRS, *The Journal of the Royal Navy Medical Service*, Spring 1984, The Medical Research Council.

Burley V.J., Blundell J.E., 'Dietary fiber and the pattern of energy intake,' in *Dietary Fiber in Health and Disease*, eds Kritchevsky D., Blomfield C., 1995, pp.243–256, Eagan Press: USA.

Burr M.L., Fehily A.M., Gilbert J.F. et al., 'Effects of changes in fat, fish, and fiber intakes on death and myocardial reinfarction: diet and reinfarction trial (DART),' *Lancet*, 1989; 2:757–761.

Calissi P.T., Jaber L.A., 'Peripheral diabetic neuropathy: current concepts in treatment,' *Ann. Pharmacotherapy*, 1995; 28:769–777.

Campbell L.V., Marmot P.E., Dyer J.A. et al., 'The high monounsaturated fat diet as a practical alternative for NIDDM,' *Diabetes Care*, 1994; 17:177–182.

Berdanier, Carolyn D. PhD, 'Mitochondrial gene expression in diabetes mellitus: effect of nutrition,' *Nutrition Reviews*, March 2001, Vol. 59, No. 3(1), 61–70.

Carter J.S., Pugh J.A., Monterrosa A., 'Noninsulin dependent diabetes mellitus in minorities in the United States,' *Ann. Intern. Med.*, 1996; 125:221–232.

Castelli W., *Arteriosclerosis*, 1996; 124:S1–S9.

Cenacchi, T. et al., 'Cognitive decline in the elderly: a double-blind, placebo-controlled multicenter study on efficacy of phosphatidylserine administration,' *Aging*, 1993; 5:123–33.

Chernow B., Alexander R., Smallridge R.C., Thompson W.R., Cook D., Beardsley D., Fink M.P., Lake R., Fletcher J.R., 'Hormonal responses to graded surgical stress,' *Arch. Intern. Med.*, 1987; 147: 1273–1278.

Cleave T.L., 'The saccharine disease,' 1974, Bristol, John Wright.

Clements R.S., 'Peripheral nerve biochemistry in diabetes,' *Clin. Physiol.*, 1985; 5:19–22.

Cooke, John, 'Defending the heart: the nitric oxide connection,' at the 10th International Symposium of Functional Medicine, Tucson, Arizona, May 2003.

Crawford M.A., 'The role of dietary fatty acids in biology: their place in the evolution of the human brain,' *Nutr. Rev.* 1992; 50:3–11.

Crawford M.A., Casperd N., Sinclair A.J., 'The long chain metabolites of linoleic and linolenic acids in liver and brains of herbivores and carnivores'. *Comp. Biochem. Physiol.* 1976; 54B:395–401.

Crawford M.A., Gale M.M., Woodford M.H., Casperd N.M., 'Comparative studies on fatty acid composition of wild and domestic meats.' *Int. J. Biochem.,* 1970; 1:295–305.

Critser, Greg, *Fat Land* (about How Americans Became the Fattest People on Earth), June 2003.

Crook, T.H. et al., 'Effects of phosphatidylserine in age-associated memory impairment,' *Neurology,* 1991; 41:644–9.

Cunnance S.C., Harbige L.S., Crawford M.A., 'The importance of energy and nutrient supply in human brain evolution,' *Nutr. Health,* 1993; 9:219–235.

Davidson M.B., 'The effect of aging on carbohydrate metabolism: a review of the English literature and a practical approach to the diagnosis of diabetes mellitus in the elderly,' *Metabolism,* 1979; 28:688–705.

Davies K., Heaney R. et al., 'Calcium Intake and Body Weight,' *J. Clin. Endocrinology and Metabolism,* 2000; 85, No. 12: 4635–4638.

Davis B.D., 'Frontiers of the biological sciences,' *Science,* 1980; 209:288.

Delargy H.J., Burley V.J., O'Sullivan K.R., Fletcher R.J., Blundell J.E., 'Effects of soluble: insoluble fiber ratios at breakfast on 24 hour pattern of dietary intake and satiety,' *Eur. J. Clin. Nutr.,* 1995; 49:754–766.

Delwaide P.J. et al., 'Double-blind, randomized controlled study of phosphatidylserine in demented subjects,' *Acta Neurol. Scand.,* 1986; 73:136–140.

Di Lorenzo C., Williams C.M., Hajnal F., Valnenzuela J.E., 'Pectin delays gastric emptying and increases satiety in obese subjects,' *Gastroenterology,* 1988; 95:1211–1215.

Diamond J., 'The double puzzle of diabetes,' *Nature,* June 5, 2003; 423: 599–602.

Dilman and Dean, 'The neuroendocrine theory of aging and degenerative disease,' The Center for Bio-Gerentology, p.26., Pensacola, Florida, 1992.

Dossey L., 'Space, time, and medicine,' Boulder, Colorado, Shambala Publications Inc., 1982.

Druckler S., 'New MI: Disorders of adrenal steroidgenesis,' *Pediatr. Clin. North Am.,* 34:1055–1066.

Duell, Dr Barton, 'Homocysteine & folate metabolism: what you eat really matters,' at 10th International Symposium on Functional Medicine, May 23, 2003, Tucson, Arizona.

Duncan M.H., Singh B.M., Wise P.H., Carter G., Alaghband–Zadeh J., 'A simple measure of Insulin Resistance,' Dept. of Chemical Pathology and Endocrinology, Charing Cross Hospital, London, in *Lancet*, 1995.

Dutta-Roy A.K., 'Insulin mediated processes in platelets, erythrocytes, and monocytes/macrophages: effects of essential fatty acid metabolism,' *Prostaglandins Leukot Essential Fatty Acids*, 1994; 48:381–388.

Ebbeling C.B., Ludwig D.S., 'Treating obesity in youth: should dietary glycemic load be a consideration?,' *Adv. Pediatr.*, 2001;48:179–212.

Echert C.D., Breskin M.W., Wise W.W., Knopp R.H., 'Association between low serum selenium and diminished visual function in diabetic women,' *Fed. Proc.*, 1985; 44:1670.

Elbein S., Chiu K., Permutt M., *The Genetic Basis of Common Disease*, 2nd edn, eds King R., Rotter J., Motulsky A., 457–480, Oxford University Press, 2002.

Emdin S.O., Dodson G.G., Cutfield J.M., Cutfield S.M., 'Rose of zinc in insulin biosynthesis. Some possible zinc-insulin interactions in the pancreatic B-cell,' *Diabetologial*, 1980; 19:172–182.

Enig M.G., Atal S., Keeney M., Sampunga J., 'Isomeric trans fatty acids in the US diet,' *J. Am. Coll. Nutr.*, 1990; 5:471–486.

Eritsland J., Deljeflot I., Abdelnoor M. et al., 'Long-term effects of n-3 fatty acids on serum lipids & glycaemic control,' *Scand. J. Clin. Lab. Invest.*, 1994; 54:73–80.

Facchini F., Coulston A.M., Reaven G.M., 'Relation between dietary vitamin intake and resistance to insulin-mediated glucose disposal in healthy volunteers'. *Am. J. Clin. Nutr.*, 1996; 63:946–949.

Fagin J.A., Ikejiri K., Levin S.R., 'Insulinotropic effects of vanadate,' *Diabetes*, 1987; 36:1448.

Ferrannini E., Balkau B., 'Insulin: in search of a syndrome,' *Diabetes*, 2002; 19:724–729.

Ferrannini E., Buzzigoli G., Bonadonna R. et al., 'Insulin Resistance in essential hyper tension,' *NEJM*, 1987; 317(6):350–8.

Ferranni E., Vichi S., Beck-Nielsen H. et al., 'European group for the study of Insulin Resistance: insulin action and age,' *Diabetes*, 1996; 45: 947–53.

Food & Agriculture Organisation paper 57—WHO and FAO Joint Consultation: 'Fats & Oils in Human Nutrition,' *Nutri. Sci. Policy*, July 1995:202–205.

Ford E.S., Giles W.H., Dietz W.H., 'Prevalence of the metabolic syndrome among US adults: findings from the Third National Health and Nutrition Examination Survey,' *JAMA*, 2002; 287:356–359.

Fore H., 'Manganese-induced hypoglycemia,' *Lancet*, 1963;1:274–275.

French S.J., Read N.W., 'Effect of guar gum on hunger & satiety after meals of differing fat content: relationship with gastric emptying.' *Am. J. Clin. Nutr.*, 1994; 59: 87–91.

Fruhbeck G., Sopena M., Martinez J.A., Salvador J., 'Nutrition, energy balance, and obesity' [article in Spanish], *Rev. Med. Univ. Navarra*, Jul–Sep 1997; 41(3):185–92.

Gissi Prevenzione Investigators, 'Dietary supplementation with n-3 polyunsaturated fatty acids and vitamin E after myocardial infarction: results of the Gissi Prevenzione trial,' *Lancet*, 1999; 354:441–453.

Goodpaster B.H., Kelley D.E., 'Role of muscle in triglyceride metabolism,' *Curr. Opin. Lipidol*, 1998; 9:231–6

Goodpaster B.H., Thaete F.L., Simoneau J-A., Kelley D.E., 'Subcutaneous abdominal fat and thigh muscle composition predict insulin sensitivity independent of visceral fat,' *Diabetes*, 1997; 46:1579–85.

Graham G.C., Placko R.P., Moralk E. et al., 'Dietary protein quality in infants and children,' *Am. J. Dis. Child*, 1970; 120:419–23.

Gray D.S., 'The clinical uses of dietary fiber,' *Am. Family Physician*, 1995; 51(2): 419–426.

Guarnieri G.F., Ranieri F., Toigo G. et al., 'Lipid-lowering effect of carnitine in chronically uremic patients treated with maintenance hemodialysis,' *Am. J. Clin. Nutr.*, 1980; 33:1489–1492.

Hackett A., Nathan I., Burgess L., 'Is a vegetarian diet adequate for children,' *Nutr. Health.*, 1998; 12(3):189–95.

Harman D., 'Free radicals and the origin, evolution, and present status of the free radical theory of aging,' *Free Radicals in Molecular Biology, Aging, and Disease*, ed. D. Armstrong et al., New York, Raven.

Haugen H.N., 'The blood concentration of thiamine in diabetes,' Scand. J. Clin. Lab. Invest., 1964; 16:260–266.

Hayashi T. et al., 'Ellagitannins from Lagerstroemia speciosa as activators of glucose transport in fat cells,' *Planta Med.*, Feb 2002; 68(2):173–5.

Henricksson, I., 'Effect of exercise on amino acid concentration in skeletal muscle and plasma,' *J. Exper. Biol.*, 1991; 160:149–165.

Herington A.C., 'Effect of zinc on insulin binding to rat adipocytes and hepatic membranes and to human placental membranes and IM–9 lymphocytes,' *Horm. Metab. Res.*, 1985; 17:328–332.

Himsworth H.P., Kerr R.B., 'Insulin-sensitive and insulin-insensitive types of diabetes mellitus,' *Clin. Sci.*, 1939; 4:119–52.

Holman R.T., Johnson S.B., Ogburn P.L., 'Deficiency of essential fatty acids and membrane fluidity during pregnancy and lactation,' *Natl. Acad. Sci. USA*, 1991; 88:4835–4839.

Holt S., Brand-Miller J.C., 'Increased insulin responses to ingested foods associated with lessened satiety,' *Appetite*, 1995; 24:43–54.

Holub B.J., 'The nutritional importance of inositol and the phosphinositides,' *NEJM*, 1992; 326:1285–1286.

Horrobin D.F., 'Fatty acid metabolism in health & disease; the role of D-6-desaturase,' *Am. J. Clin. Nutr.*, 1993; 57(suppl.):732S–737S.

Horrobin D.F., 'Abnormal membrane concentrations of 20 and 22-carbon essential fatty acids: a common link between risk factors and coronary and peripheral vascular disease?,' *Prostaglandins Leukot Essent. Fatty Acids*, 1995; 53:85–396.

Horrobin D.F., 'Essential fatty acid (EFA) metabolism in patients with diabetic neuropathy,' *Prostaglandins Leukot Essential Fatty Acids*, 1997; 57:256 (abstr.).

Hotamisligil G.S., Spiegelman B.M., 'Tumor necrosis factor alpha: a key component of the obesity–diabetes link,' *Diabetes*, 1994; 43:1271–1278.

Humphrys, J., *The Great Food Gamble*, Hodder & Stoughton, 2001.

Hyams J.S., Carey D.E., 'Corticosteroids and growth,' *J. Paeditr.*, 1988; 113: 249–254.

Jacob, S., Henrikson E.J., Ruus P. et al., 'The radical scavenger a-lipoic acid enhances insulin sensitivity in patients with NIDDM: A placebo controlled trial,' presented at Oxidants and Antioxidants in Biology, Santa Barbara, CA, February 26–March 1, 1997.

Jacob, S., Henriskon E.J., Schiemann A.L. et al., 'Enhancement of glucose disposal in patients with type 2 diabetes by alpha-lipoic acid,' *Arzneimittel-Forsuchung Drug Research*, 1995; 45:872–874.

Jain S.K., Lim G., 'Lipoic acid (LA) decreases protein glycation and increases (Na++K+) and Ca++-ATPases activities in high glucose (G)-treated red blood cells (RBC),' *Free Radical Biology & Medicine*, 1998; 25:S94, Abstract #268.

James P., Norum K., Rosenberg I., 'The nutritional role of fat,' *Meeting Summary Nut. Rev.*, 1992; 50:68–70.

Jenkins D.J.A., Wolever T.M.S., Leeds A.R., Gassull M.A., Haisman P., Dilawari J., Goff D.V., Metz G.L., Alberti K.G.M.M., 'Dietary fibers, fiber analogies, & glucose tolerance: importance of viscosity,' *Br. Med. J.*, 1978; 1: 1392–1394.

Jeppesen L.L. et al., 'Decreased serum testosterone in men with acute ischemic stroke,' *Arterioscler. Thromb. Vac. Biol.*, 1996; 16:749–54.

Kahn B.B., Rosetti L., 'Type 2 diabetes—who is conducting the orchestra?' *Nature Genetics*, 1998; 20:223–225.

Kakuda T., Sakane I., Takihara T., Ozaki Y., Takeuchi H., Kuroyanagi M., 'Hypoglycemic effect of extracts from Lagerstroemia speciosa L. leaves in genetically diabetic KK-AY mice,' *Biosci. Biotechnol. Biochem.*, Feb 1996; 60(2):204–8.

Keen II., Mattock M.D., 'Complications of diabetes mellitus: role of essential fatty acids,' in Horrobin D.F. (ed.), *Omega-6 Essential Fatty Acid. Pathophysiology & Roles in Clinical Medicine*, Wiley-Liss, New York, 1990:447–455.

Khan M.I., Read N.W., 'The effect of duodenal lipid infusions upon gastric pressure and sensory responses to balloon distension,' *Gastroeneterology*, 1992; 102: 467.

King H., Aubert R., Herman W., *Diabetes Care*, 1998; 21:1414–1431.

Konrad T, Vivina P, Kusterer K, et al., 'a-lipoic acid treatment decreases serum lactate and pyruvate concentrations and improves glucose effectiveness in lean and obese patients with type 2 diabetes,' *Diabetes Care*, 1999; 22:280–287.

Kozlovsky A.S., Moser P.B., Reiser S., Anderson R.A. 'Effects of diets high in simple sugars on chromium urinary losses,' *Metabolism*, 1986; 35:515–518.

Krajcovicova-Kudlackova M., Simoncic R., Bederova A., 'Risks and advantages of the vegetarian diet,' *Cas. Lek. Cesk.*, Dec. 3 1997; 136(23):715–9.

Kreiger D.T., 'Rhythms of ACTH and corticosteroid secretion in health and disease and their experimental modification,' *J. Steroid Biochem.*, 1975; 6:785–791.

Kruszynska Y.T., Olefsky J.M., 'Cellular and molecular mechanisms of non-insulin dependent diabetes mellitus,' *J. Invest. Med.*, 1996; 44(8):413–28.

Lancet, May 8, 1999; 353:1586–7.

Laudat M.H., Cerdos S., Fournier C., Guinban D., Guithaume B., Luton J.P., *J. Clin. Endocrinol. Metab.*, 1988; 66:343.

Leproult R., et al., 'Sleep loss results in an elevation of cortisol levels the next evening,' *Sleep*, 1997; 20:865–70.

Lifshitz F., Moak S.A., Wapnir R.A., 'Folic acid in the prevention of fasting induced hypoglycemia,' *Pediatr. Res.*, 1977; 11:518.

Lillioja S., Mott D., Spraul M., et al., 'Insulin resistance as precursor of non-insulin dependent diabetes mellitus. Prospective studies of Pima Indians,' *NEJM*, 1993; 29:1988–1992.

Lissner L., Bengtsson C., Kristansson K., Wedel H., 'Fasting insulin in relation to subsequent blood pressure changes and hypertension in women,' *Hypertension*, 1992; 20:797–801.

Liu F., Kim J., Li Y., Liu X., Li J., Chen X., 'An extract of Lagerstroemia speciosa L. has insulin-like glucose uptake-stimulatory and adipocyte differentiation-inhibitory activities in 3T3-L1 cells,' *J. Nutr.*, Sept. 2001; 131(9):2242–7.

Liu S., Willett W.C., Stampfer M,J,, et al., 'A prospective study of dietary glycemic load, carbohydrate intake, and risk of coronary heart disease in US women,' *Am. J. Clin. Nutr.*, 2000; 71:1455–1461.

Lord, R.S., Bralley, A.J., 'Polyunsaturated fatty acid-induced antioxidant deficiency,' *Integrative Medicine*, 2003; 1(1):38–44.

Luo J., Rizkalla S.W., Boillot J., et al., 'Dietary (n-3) polyunsaturated fatty acids improve adipocyte insulin action and glucose metabolism in insulin-resistance rats: relation to membrane fatty acids,' *J. Nutr.*, 1996; 126: 1951–1958.

MacGregor A.B., *Annals of the Royal College of Surgeons of England*, 1964; 34:179.

Maebashi M., Kawamura N., Sato M., Immura A., Yoshinaga K., 'Lipid-lowering effects of carnitine in patients with Type IV hypertriglyceri-daemia,' *Lancet*, 1978; 805–807.

McAuley K.A., Williams S.M., Mann J.I., et al., 'Diagnosing Insulin Resistance in the general population,' *Diabetes Care*, 2001; 24:460–464.

McKeigue P.M., Shah B., Marmot M.G., 'Relation of central obesity and insulin resistance with high diabetes prevalence and cardiovascular risk in South Asians,' *Lancet*, 1991; 337:382–386.

Mensink and Karan, *Lancet*, 1987; 1:122–125.

Mensink and Katan, *NEJM*, 1990; 323:439–445.

Mertz, W. 'Chromium in human nutrition: a review,' *J. Nutr.*, 1993; 123: 626–633.

Millward D.J., 'The nutritional value of plant-based diets in relation to human amino acid and protein requirements,' *Proc. Nutr. Soc.*, May 1999; 58(2):249–60.

Monteleone, P., et al., 'Blunting chronic PS administration of the stress-induced activation of the hypothalamo-pituitary-adrenal axis in healthy men,' *Eur. J. Clin. Pharmacol.*, 1992; 41:385–8.

Murakami C., Myoga K., Kasai R., Ohtani K., Kurokawa T., Ishibashi S., Dayrit F., Padolina W.G., Yamasaki K., 'Screening of plant constituents for effect on glucose transport activity in Ehrlich ascites tumor cells,' *Chem. Pharm. Bull. (Tokyo)*, Dec 1993; 41(12):2129–31.

Murray, M. ND, *The Healing Power of Foods*, Prima Publishing, 1993.

Nantel G. PhD, 'Glycemic carbohydrate: an international perspective,' *Nutrition Reviews*, May 2003; (II)S34–S39.

National Research Council, Commission on Diet & Health 1989, National Academic Press, page 7.

Nee J.V., 'Diabetes mellitus: a "thrifty" genotype rendered detrimental by "progress",' *Am. J. Hum. Genetics*, 1962; 14:353–362.

Nigeon C.J., Lanes R.L., *Adrenal Cortex: hypo and hyperfunction. Paediatrci Endocrinology. A Clinical Guide*, second edition, Marcel Decker Inc., New York, 1990, pp.333–352.

O'Dea K., 'Traditional diet & food preferences of Australian Aboriginal hunter-gatherers,' *Phil. Trans. Royal Soc. London B.*, 1991; 334:233–241.

Oliver M.F., 'Doubts about preventing coronary heart disease,' *BMJ*, 1992; 304:393–394.

Ong K.K., Dunger D.B., 'Perinatal growth failure: the road to obesity, insulin resistance, and cardiovascular disease in adults,' *Best Practice Res. Clin. Endocrinol. Metab.*, 2002; 16:191–207.

Packer L., Witt E.H., Tritschler H.J., 'Alpha-lipoic acid as a biological antioxidant,' *Free Radical Biology & Medicine*, 1995; 19:227–250.

Pan D.A., Lillioja S., Kriketos A.D., et al., 'Skeletal muscle triglyceride levels are inversely related to insulin action,' *Diabetes*, 1997; 46(6):9983–8.

Pan D.A., Lillioja S., Milner M.R., et al., 'Skeletal muscle membrane lipid composition is related to adiposity & insulin action,' *J. Clin. Invest.*, 1995; 96:2802–2808.

Paolisso, G., Di Maro, G., Galzerano, D., et al., 'Pharmacological doses of vitamin E and insulin action in elderly subjects,' *Am. J. Clin. Nutr.*, 1994; 59:1291–1296.

Pasquali R., Vicennati V., 'Activity of the hypothalamic-pituitary-adrenal axis in different phenotypes,' *Int. J. Obes. Relat. Metab. Disord.*, Jun. 2000; 24 Suppl. 2:S47–9.

Peerenboom H., Keck E., 'The significance of magnesium in medicine. (I) Biological function, homeostasis, ingestion, and excretion,' [author's transl., article in German], *MMW Munch Med. Wochenschr.*, September 26, 1980; 122(39):1325–7.

Peponis V., Papathanasiou M., Kapranou A., Magkou C., Tyligada A., Melidonis A., Drosos T., Sitaras N.M., 'Protective role of oral antioxidant supplementation in ocular surface of diabetic patients,' *Br. J. Ophthalmol.*, Dec. 2002; 86(12):1369–73.

Pinto R.J., 'Risk factors for coronary heart disease in Asian Indians: clinical implications for prevention of coronary heart disease,' *Indian J. Med. Sci.*, Feb. 1998; 52(2):49–54.

Pressman A., *The GSH Phenomenon*, St. Martin's Press, New York, 1997.

Raben A., Due Jensen N., Marckmann P., Sandstrom B., Astrup A., 'Spontaneous weight loss during 11 weeks' ad libitum intake of a low fat/high fiber diet in young, normal weight subjects,' *Int. J. Obesity*, 1995; 19: 916–923.

Raber, J., 'Detrimental effects of chronic hypothalamic-pituitary adrenal axis activation. From obesity to memory deficits,' *Mol. Neruobiol.*, Aug 1998; (1):1–22.

Ravelli G.-P., Stain Z.A., Susser M.W., 'Obesity in young men after famine exposure in utero and early infancy,' *NEJM*, 1976; 295:349–353.

Ravussin E., Bogardus C., 'Energy expenditure in the obese: is there a thrifty gene?,' *Infusiostherapie*, 1990; 76:108–112.

Read G.F., Walker R.F., Wilson D.W., Griffiths K., 'Steroid analysis in saliva for the assessment of endocrine function,' *Ann. Ny. Acad. Sci.*, 1990; 595: 260–274.

Read N.W., French S.J., Cunningham K.M., 'The role of the gut in regulating food intake in man,' *Nutr. Rev.*, 1994; 52:1–10.

Reaven, G.M., 'Role of Insulin Resistance in human disease,' *Diabetes*, 1988; 37:1595–1607.

Reaven G.M., Reaven E.P., 'Effect of age on various aspects of glucose metabolism,' *Mol. Cell. Biochem.*, 1980; 31:37–47.

Reaven G.M., Reaven E.P., 'Age, glucose intolerance, and noninsulin-dependent diabetes mellitus,' *J. Am. Geriatr. Soc.*, 1985; 33:286–90.

Reaven G., Strom, T.K., Fox B., *Syndrome X The Silent Killer*, Fireside Books, New York, NY, 2000, p.18.

Renaud, S.V. MD, PhD, Lanzmann-Petithory MD, 'Dietary fats & coronary heart disease pathogenesis,' *Current Atherosclerosis Reports*, 2002; 4:419–424.

Ritter M.M., Richter W.O., 'Effects of a vegetarian life style on health' [article in German], *Fortschr. Med.*, 10 Jun. 1995; 113(16):239–42.

Rodriguez Jimenez J., Rodriguez J.R., Gonzalez M.J., 'Indicators of anxiety and depression in subjects with different kinds of diet: vegetarians and omnivores' [in Spanish], *Bol. Asoc. Med. P. R.*, Apr–Jun 1998; 90(4–6):58–68.

Rosmond R., M.D. PhD, et al., 'Alterations in the hypothalamic pituitary adrenal axis in metabolic syndromes,' December 2001; 491–497.

Ross, J., *The Diet Cure*, Michael Joseph, 2000, p.162.

Roth, J.L., Mobarhan S., Clohisy M., 'The metabolic syndrome: where are we and where do we go?,' *Nutrition Reviews*, 2002; 60(11):335–337.

Rowley K.G., Best J.D., McDermott R., Green E.A., Piers L.S., O'Dea K., 'Insulin resistance syndrome in Australian aboriginal people,' *Clin. Exp. Pharmacol. Physiol.*, Sep–Oct 1997; 24(9–10):776–81.

Salmeron J. et al., *JAMA*, 1997; 277:472–477.

Salmeron J., Manson J.E., Stampfer M.J., et al., 'Dietary fiber, glycemic load, and risk of noninsulin-dependent diabetes mellitus in women,' *JAMA*, 1997; 277:472–477

Salmeron J., Ascherio A., Rimm E.B., et al., 'Dietary fiber, glycemic load, and risk of NIDDM in men,' *Diabetes Care*, 1997; 20:545–550.

Salway J.G., Whitehead L., Finnegan J.A., Karunanayaka A., Burnett D., Payne R.B., 'Effect of myo-inositol on peripheral-nerve function in diabetes,' *Lancet*, 1978; 1282–1284.

Sandoval-Chacon, M., et al. 'Antiinflammatory actions of cat's claw: the role of NF-kB,' *Aliment. Pharmacol. Ther.*, 1998; 12:1279–1289.

Saris W.H.M, MD, PhD. 'Glycemic carbohydrate and body weight regulation,' *Nutrition Reviews*, May 2003; (II)S10–S11.

Sarkinnen E., Schwab U., Niskanen L., et al., 'The effects of monounsaturated-fat enriched diet and polyunsaturated-fat enriched diet on lipid and glucose metabolism in subjects with impaired glucose tolerance,' *Eur. J. Clin. Nutr.*, 1996; 60:592–598.

Schlosser, E., *Fast Food Nation*, Penguin Books, 2001.

Schmidt N.A., *Issues Compr. Pediatr. Nurtr.*, 1998; 20(3)183–90.

Science, September 22, 2000; 289:2122–2125.

Secher K., 'The bearing of the ascorbic acid content of the blood on the course of the blood sugar curve,' *Acta. Med. Scand.*, 1942; 60:255–265.

Seelig M.S., 'Consequences of magnesium deficiency on the enhancement of stress reactions; preventive and therapeutic implications. (A Review),' *J. Am. Coll. Nutr.*, 1994; 13(5):429–446.

Shah M., Garg A. ,'High fat and high carbohydrate diets and energy balance,' *Diabetes Care*, 1996; 19:1142–1152.

Shapiro J., et al., 'Testosterone and other anabolic steroids as cardiovascular drugs,' *Am. J. Ther.*, 1999; 6:167–74.

Shulman G.I., Rothman D.L., Jue T., et al., 'Quantitation of muscle glycogen synthesis in normal subjects and subjects with noninsulin dependent diabetes by 13C nuclear magnetic resonance spectroscopy,' *NEJM*, 1990; 322(4):223–8.

Simon, D., et al., 'Association between plasma total testosterone and cardiovascular risk factors in healthy adult men: The Telecom Study,' *J. Clin. Endocrinol. Metab.*, 1997; 82:682–5.

Sinclair A.J., Gibson R., eds., 'Essential fatty acids and eicosanoids: invited papers from the Third International Conference,' *Campaign*, IL: AOCS Press; 1993.

Skarfors E.T., Lithell O., Selinus I., 'Risk factors for the development of hypertension: a ten year longitudinal study in middle-aged men,' *Journal of Hypertension*, 1991; 9:217–223.

Solyst, J.T., Michaelis I.V., O.E., Reiser S., Ellwood K.C., Prather E.S., 'Effect of dietary sucrose in humans on blood uric acid, phosphorous, fructose, and lactic acid responses to a sucrose load,' *Nutr. Metabol.*, 1980; 24:182.

Stevens J., Levitsky D.A., VanSoest P.L., Robertson J.B., Kalkwark H.J., Roe D.A., 'Effect of psyllium gum and wheat bran on spontaneous energy intake,' *Am. J. Clin. Nutr.*, 1987; 46:812–817.

Storlien L.H., Jenkins A.B., Chisholm D.J., et al., 'Influence of dietary fat composition on development of insulin resistance in rats,' *Diabetes*, 1991; 40:280–289.

Storlien L.H., Pan D.A., Kriketos A.D., et al., 'Skeletal muscle membrane lipids and insulin resistance,' *Lipids*, 1996; 31:S262–S265.

Stuhlinger et al., *JAMA*, 2002, 287(11):1420–1426.

Suzuki Y., Unno T., Ushitani M., Hayashi K., Kakuda T., 'Antiobesity activity of extracts from Lagerstroemia speciosa L. leaves on female KK-Ay mice,' *J. Nutr. Sci. Vitaminol.* (Tokyo), Dec 1999; 45(6):791–5.

Swendseid M.E., Kopple J.D., 'L-Histidine is an essential amino acid,' *Infusionsther Klin. Ernahr.*, Jun. 1975; 2(3):203–7.

Szanto S., Yudkin J., 'The effects of dietary sucrose on blood lipids, serum insulin, platelet adhesiveness, and bony weight in human volunteers,' *Postgrad. Med. J.*, 1969; 45:602–7.

Szanto S., Yudkin J., Kakkar V.V., 'Sugar intake, serum insulin, and platelet adhesiveness in men with and without peripheral vascular disease,' *Postgrad. Med. J.*, 1969; 45:608–11.

Szathmary E.J.E., 'Noninsulin dependent diabetes mellitus among aboriginal North Americans,' *Ann. Rev. Anth.*, 194; 23:457–482.

Tataranni P.A., Baier L.J., Paolisso G., et al., 'Role of lipids in development of noninsulin dependent diabetes mellitus: lessons learned from Pima Indians,' *Lipids*, 1996; 337:382–386.

Taylor S.R., McLennan S.M., 'The continental crust: its composition and evolution,' Oxford, Blackwell; 1985.

Tessari P., 'Changes in Protein, Carbohydrate, and Fat metabolism with Aging: Possible Role of Insulin,' *Nutrition Reviews*, 2000; 58(1):11–19.

Teufel N.I., 'Nutrient characteristics of southwest Native American precontact diets,' *J. Nutr. Environ. Med.*, 1996; 6:273–284.

The British Heart Foundation (BHF) Statistics, 2003.

The Colgan Institute, San Diego, 1997, in Colgan, Dr. M., *The Right Protein for Muscle & Strength*, Progressive Health Series, Apple Publishing, 1998.

'The Metabolic Syndrome,' *Journal of Internal Medicine*, 1994; 236(suppl . 736):13–22.

The Quebec Heart Study—Circulation 1997; 95:73.

Thorburn A.W., Gumbiner B., Bulacan F., et al., 'Intracellular glucose oxidation and glycogen synthase activity are reduced in noninsulin-dependent (type II) diabetes independent of impaired glucose uptake,' *J. Clin. Invest.*, 1990; 85:522–9

Tiblin G., et al., 'The pituitary-gonadal axis and health in elderly men: a study of men born in 1913,' *Diabetes*, 1996; 45:1605–10.

Velussi M., Cernigoi A.M., De Monte A. et al., 'Long term (12 months) treatment with an antioxidant drug (silymarin) is effective in hyperinsulinemia, exogenous insulin need, and malondialdehyde levels in cirrhotic diabetic patients,' *Journal of Hepatology,* 1997; 26:871–879.

Vining R.F., McGinley R.A., Maksvytis J.J., Ho K.Y., *Ann. Clin. Biochem.,* 1983, 20:329–35

Waugh W., 'Orthomolecular medical use of L-Citrulline for vasoprotection, relaxative smooth muscle tone & cell protection,' United States Patent No. 5, 874, 471, 1999.

Waught W., Daeschner W., Files B., McConnel M., Stranjord S., 'Oral citrulline as Arginine precursor,' *J. Nat. Med. Assoc.,* 2001.

Weaver C.M., Heaney R., Shils M. et al., eds, *Modern Nutrition in Health and Disease,* 9th edition, 1999, Lippincott, Williams and Wilkins, p.141–143.

Wedepohl K.H., 'The composition of the continental crust,' *Geochim Cosmochim Acta,* 1995; 59:1217–1232.

Wendorf M., 'Archaeology and the "thrifty" noninsulin dependent diabetes mellitus (NIDDM) genotype,' *Adv. Perit. Dial.,* 1992; 8:201–7.

Wilkinson J.F., 'Diabetes mellitus and pernicious anemia,' *Br. Med. J.,* 1963; 1:676–677.

Willett W. MD, Lecture at the Tenth International Symposium on Functional Medicine: The Heart on Fire, Tucson, Arizona, May 25, 2003.

Willett W. MD, 'Improving CVD risk: an epidemiological perspective,' May 25, 2003, 10th International Symposium on Functional Medicine, Tucson, Arizona.

Willett W. MD, Stampfer, M., MD, 'Rebuilding the food pyramid,' *Scientific American,* December 17, 2002.

Williams, Dr. Roger, *The Wonderful World Within You: Your Inner Nutritional Environment,* 1977.

Windmueller H., Spaeth A., 'Source & fate of circulating citrulline,' *Am. J. Physiol.,* 1981; 241:E473.

Wolf G., 'Adult type 2 diabetes induced by intrauterine growth retardation,' *Nutrition Reviews,* May 2003; 61(5):176–179.

Yajnik, Chittaranja S. MD, 'The Insulin Resistance epidemic in India: fetal origins, later lifestyle, or both?,' *Nutrition Reviews,* Vol. 59, No. 1 (part I), January 2001.

Yamamoto T. DDS, PhD, 'Brain mechanisms of sweetness & palatability of sugars,' *Nutrition Reviews,* May 2003; (II)S5–S9.

Young V.R., et al., 'A theoretical basis for increasing current estimates of the amino acid requirements in adult man with experimental support,' *Am.*

J. Clin. Nutr., 1989; 50:80–92.

Yudkin J., 'Dietary factors in atherosclerosis,' *Lipids,* 1978; 13:370–2.

Yudkin, J., 'Diet & coronary heart disease: why blame fat?,' *J. of Royal Soc. of Med.,* Sept 1992, p.5.

Zemel M.B., Shi H., Greer B., Dirienzo D., Zemel P.C., 'Regulation of adiposity by dietary calcium,' *The FASEB Journal,* 2000; 14:1132–1138.

Ziegler D., Gries F.A., 'Alpha-lipoic acid in the treatment of diabetic peripheral and cardiac autonomic neuropathy,' *Diabetes,* 1997; 46(S):S62–S66.

Ziegler D., Schatz H., Conrad F. et al., 'Effects of treatment with the antioxidant alpha-lipoic acid on cardiac autonomic neuropathy in NIDDM patients,' *Diabetes Care,* 1997; 20:369–373.

Zimmet P. in *The Medical Challenge: Complex Traits,* eds Fischer E. and Moller G., 55–110, Piper Munich, 1997.

Zimmet P., Alberti K., Shaw J., *Nature,* 2001; 414:782–787.

Zmuda J.M. et al., 'Longitudinal relation between endogenous testosterone and cardiovascular disease risk factors in middle-aged men. A 13 yr followup of former multiple risk factor intervention trial participants,' *Am. J. Epidemiol.,* 1997; 146:609–17.

Bibliography

Batmanghelidj, Dr. F., *Your Body's Many Cries for Water*, Global Health Solutions, 1995.

Beverley, Bernard and Fairhurst, Arthur, *Protein and Amino Acids*, Sports Publications & Marketing Ltd., 1987.

Challem, Jack, Berkson, Burton MD and Smith, Melissa Diane, *Syndrome X*, John Wiley & Sons Inc., New York, 2000.

Colgan, Michael PhD, *The Right Protein for Muscle and Strength*, Progressive Health Series by Apple Publishing Company Ltd., Vancouver, 1998.

Erasmus, Udo, *Fats that Heal, Fats that Kill*, Alive Books, 3rd printing 1989.

Galland, Dr. Leo, *The Four Pillars of Healing*, Random House, 1997.

Golan, Ralph MD, *Optimal Wellness*, Ballantine Books, New York, 1995.

Kenton, Leslie, *The X Factor Diet*, Vermilion, London, 2002.

Levine, Stephen PhD and Kidd, Parris PhD, *Antioxidant Adaptation*, Allergy Research Group, 4th printing 2001.

Linder, Maria (ed.), *Nutritional Biochemistry and Metabolism*, Appleton & Lange, 1991.

Murray, Michael ND, *The Healing Power of Foods*, Prima Publishing, California, 1993.

O'Riordan, J.L.H., Malan P.G. and Gould R.P. (eds), *Essentials of Endocrinology*, Blackwell Scientific Publications, London, 2nd edition, 1988.

Pottenger, Francis M., Jr, MD, *Pottenger's Cats—A Study in Nutrition*, Price-Pottenger Nutrition Foundation, 2nd edition 1995 (1st edition 1983).

Pressman, Alan, *The GSH Phenomenon*, St. Martin's Press, New York, 1997.

Price, Weston DDS, *Nutrition and Physical Degeneration*, Price-Pottenger Nutrition Foundation, 6th edition 1997 (1st edition 1939).

Reaven, Gerald MD, Strom, Terry Kristen MBA and Fox, Barry PhD, *Syndrome X The Silent Killer*, Fireside, New York, 2001.

Ridley, Matt, *Genome*, Fourth Estate Ltd, London, 2000.

Ross, Julia, *The Diet Cure*, Michael Joseph, London, 2000.

Schwarzbein, Diana and Brown, Marilyn, *The Schwarzbein Principle II*, Health Communications Inc, Florida, 2002.

Sears, Barry PhD, *The Zone*.

Smythies, John MD, *Every Person's Guide to Antioxidants*, Rutgers University Press, New Jersey, 1998.

Williams, Dr. Roger, *The Wonderful World Within You*, Bantam Books, 1977.

Wills, Eric D., *Biochemical Basis of Medicine*, John Wright & Sons, 1985.

Wunderlich, Ray C., Jr., MD, *Sugar and Your Health*, Good Health Publications, Florida, 1982.

Index